Change for the Better

What comes to your mind when you think of menopause? (Perhaps you just avoid thinking about it at all!) Hot flashes...osteoporosis...depression...weight gain ... are all associated with change of life. As a result, most women dread this phase of their lives.

Dr. Orene Schoenfeld is approaching menopause. Beverly Bush Smith has experienced it. They see this not as a mid-life crisis, but as one of the natural, biological processes, which include puberty and childbirth. In *Change for the Better,* they combine experience and expertise to present the facts about menopause and dispel the fears. This compassionate, insightful book will help you prepare for change of life and prevent such medical problems as cardiovascular disease and breast cancer. You'll also learn how to cope with the physical symptoms and how to ease emotional turmoil through faith. This practical book of hope enables you to anticipate the freedoms of menopause.

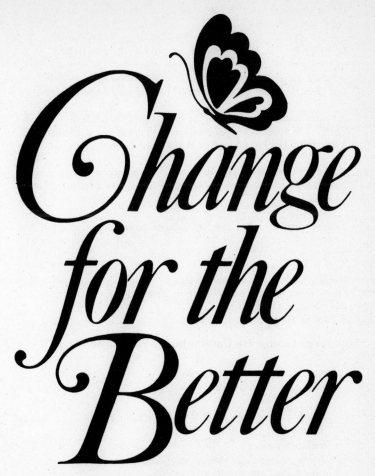

Change
for the
Better

Orene V. Schoenfeld, M.D.
and Beverly Bush Smith

**Power
Books**

FLEMING H. REVELL COMPANY
OLD TAPPAN, NEW JERSEY

Medical illustrations adapted from:
Ellen Going Jacobs and William E. Loechel
Wayne State University
School of Medicine

Library of Congress Cataloging-in-Publication Data

Schoenfeld, Orene.
    Change for the better.

    Smith's name appears first on the earlier edition.
    Bibliography: p.
    Includes index.
    1. Menopause. 2. Menopause — Psychological aspects.
I. Smith, Beverly Bush. II. Title.
RG186.S65   1988   612'.665   87-32409
ISBN 0-08007-5267-8

Copyright © 1986 by Orene V. Schoenfeld and Beverly Bush Smith.
Fleming H. Revell Company
Old Tappan, New Jersey
Printed in the United States of America

DEDICATION

This book is dedicated
to our husbands,
Dean and Bob,
who have been
so supportive to us
throughout the writing
of the book.

Orene and Beverly

CONTENTS

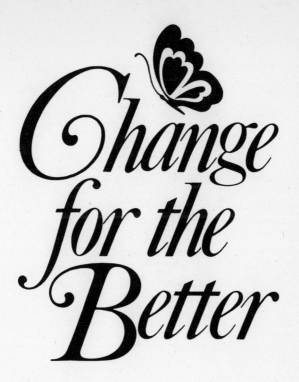

Change
for the
Better

Chapter One

CHANGE FOR THE BETTER

"If you're gonna have your change of life, you're gonna do it right now!" Archie Bunker once commanded his wife, Edith, in an episode of Norman Lear's classic TV series, "All in the Family."

"I'm gonna give you just thirty seconds. Now, come on. Change!" he demanded.[1]

If only it were that easy. And that quick!

Menopause: Half our population has either experienced it or will in the future. In the 1980 census, there were thirty-two million women in the United States of menopausal age, that is, over fifty years old, so we are talking about a good percentage of our population. Why, then, haven't we heard or learned more about this time of change? Why are we so reluctant to talk about it?

Although seventy-five percent of menopausal women have one or more bothersome symptoms, only twenty-five percent seek medical attention for their problems. In fact, for years this time of transition seemed virtually untouched by all the trends to "tell it like it is" and to "feel free to be what you are." Norman Lear was far ahead of his time when he tackled the subject on family television in 1971.

Despite the reluctance to talk about it, menopause has been with us since women lived long enough to pass into a nonreproductive state. References to menopause date back to the early centuries, and we even find biblical allusions to Sarah's personality change in her later years.

The first medical records classified menopause as a disease of social stress. Only in the past thirty years have physicians found that administration of the hormone estrogen can reverse many of these symptoms. Yet menopause for many women is still clouded with myth, muddied by controversy, and shrouded in secrecy. It's only beginning to come out of the closet.

Moreover, many women, ostrich-style, don't even want to think about it until they get there. They have no idea that as early as age thirty-five, they should be preparing for this major event in their lives, just as many of them prepared for childbirth using such approaches as the Lamaze method. In fact, Dr. Morris Notelovitz, director of the Center for Climacteric Studies in Gainesville, Florida, says, "We need a Lamaze of middle age."

Meanwhile, millions of women who are "there" face a time of adjustment, which is the mirror image of the menarche (the onset of menstruation). Remember those emotional peaks and valleys, the sudden tears, the feelings that no one understood, the times your family said you were "impossible"?

There is, of course, an enormous individual variation in the experience. Many of us breeze through and congratulate ourselves on having the right attitude. Others truly suffer and wonder, "What's wrong with me?" While many of us manage to cope with physical symptoms, such as hot flashes, insomnia, and low energy, at the same time we may feel overwhelmed by the emotions that sometimes accompany menopause: shame, fear, depression, confusion, loneliness, anger, a feeling that we are ugly and undesirable.

The authors of this book, Dr. Orene Schoenfeld and Beverly Bush Smith, understand these physical and emotional symptoms. The former brings to the book the ten-year experience of a gynecologist practicing in Gainesville, Florida, plus the anticipation of a woman looking forward to menopause, while the latter has already passed through it. "How I wish I'd had a gentle, empathetic physician at my side to guide and inform me when I experienced these complex midlife changes," Bev says. "I'm sure I'd have dealt with them far more gracefully if I'd truly understood what was happening to my body."

For instance, the most difficult time for Bev was not menopause itself, although she experienced hot flashes and other specific symptoms. It was during her forties, when she began flooding on the second day of each period and often felt as though she walked such a delicate emotional tightrope that the tiniest misstep might catapult her into complete chaos. Bev realizes now that these difficulties were probably the result of premenopausal hormone changes.

Later, after menopause, she told her internist about the vaginal discomfort she would experience during intercourse. He waited until his nurse left the room, pulled up his chair, and almost whispered, "Now, about having relations. Plenty of lubricant." Then he was gone before Bev could tell him she'd tried that!

Another problem arose six years after her last period, when her doctor strongly recommended that she begin estrogen-progesterone treatment because he felt she was in the at-risk group for osteoporosis. Bev was totally surprised, and not at all delighted, to experience a period after the first month of treatment. She needed to weigh the benefits of the hormones against the disadvantages.

Only when Bev began her own research, and finally to work with Orene Schoenfeld, did she truly find the information she needed to make a wise decision and to understand the earlier problems. Orene and Beverly have collaborated to write this book to give you the knowledge to help you cope better and, even more than that, to experience a satisfying, well-prepared passage.

Information. That's what so many of us find lacking at this time of life. No wonder so many women view menopause with such a fearful mixture of emotions!

It's our prayer that, with Bev's 20/20 hindsight and Orene's professional expertise, we can give you practical information so that you will be informed and ready. Then you can see menopause, not as the end of the world, but as an era of life which brings new freedom and zest.

We are striving for a book that is accurate from a medical standpoint and will also provide a coping mechanism for the woman of faith, a book that may be used both as a guide and as an inspiration.

We hope, too, that as you read you will begin to view aging, not as a crisis, but as an ongoing process which begins with birth and extends to death, embracing many rites of passage, such as puberty, childbirth, and menopause. Each has its degree of discomfort, each its immense rewards. We trust that we will dispel some negative feelings and fears as we show you the fallacies of many of the old wives'—and old husbands'—tales.

The last five years have produced a veritable explosion of information to keep women healthier and happier, as an increasing number of physicians focus their research on this time of life. What a contrast this focus is to just eight years ago, when a lecturing gynecologist patly stated her solution to the problems of menopause: "Drink a glass of milk and walk around the block"! How different it is from the days when an endocrinologist insisted that estrogen had no effect on the body's bony metabolism! In all of history, you couldn't have picked a better time to anticipate or participate in the menopausal years.

Since knowledge is the beginning of freedom, we will begin by clarifying just what happens to the body during menopause and afterwards. If you feel as if you're in medical school during this first chapter, don't be discouraged. The rest of the book will apply this knowledge to the everyday situations you are experiencing. We'll examine the physical symptoms and what can be done about them. We'll discuss a woman's sex life during and after menopause. We'll suggest some preventive measures you can begin using as early as age thirty-five. We'll talk about attitudes—not just our own, but men's, society's, and other cultures'—so we can understand the subtle innuendoes which lead women to fear the change of life.

Finally, we'll look to the Great Physician, who can help us through these years in a way that neither we, in our own strength, nor our doctors, in all their wisdom, can.

Just as we are now freed from the irrational fears and myths of childbirth, we can approach menopause with an informed confidence and optimism. Even if there should be some dark times, there's light at the end of the tunnel.

Chapter Two

WHAT IS MENOPAUSE?

"I feel like there's a war going on inside of me," a patient with pronounced menopausal symptoms once declared to Orene. "What's actually happening?" she asked.

A younger woman, hearing of the genesis of this book, exclaimed, "Good! I want a clear explanation of what menopause actually is, just like I had about childbirth."

Menopause is medically defined as the cessation of menstruation. The average age of menopause is steadily rising; now in this country, it is fifty-one. Most American women will experience menopause between the ages of forty and the early fifties. However, we all know that the process is simply not a single event which happens in one day, or even two. We can't just "Change!" and be done with our "change of life," as Archie Bunker insisted.

THE CLIMACTERIC

A much more accurate name for this entire period of transition is "climacteric." (The dictionary pronunciation is cly-mak'-ter-ik, but frequently we also hear the word accented on the third syllable.) This term, which may at first seem a bit technical is actually quite descriptive. It's rooted in the Greek *klimakter*, meaning the steps of a staircase. The implication then seems to be: a means of access to a point that is higher and, in some ways, better.

Certainly the word *climacteric* clearly defines a very gradual transformation that begins at about age thirty-five and ends at sixty-five. It can be viewed as the reverse or mirror image of puberty. In your preteens, your body began to change in preparation for the onset of menstruation and the maturing of your reproductive system. Now your body changes from a reproductive to a nonreproductive mode, and menstruation ceases. It is a very progressive modulation over a number of years.

The climacteric can be divided into three stages: the *perimenopause* (from the beginning of ovarian decline, age thirty-five to fifty or so), the *menopause* (at roughly age fifty-one), and the *postmenopause* (from menopause to the time symptoms cease, about age sixty-five).

Neither the climacteric nor the menopause itself is an illness, any more than puberty is an illness or a disease. In fact, the term, "ovarian failure," which some doctors use to explain these changes, seems exaggerated. Why should the medical literature term the postmenopausal woman "estrogen deficient" when we don't consider the prepubertal child as "suffering from estrogen deprivation"? The menopausal woman has not failed; she has simply passed from one stage to another.

The end of reproduction is a normal part of a woman's life, one which can give us more zest and freedom in our later years. It's curious that of all God's creatures, female human beings are the only species that continues to live and remain productive after their ovaries cease to be reproductive.

Of course, there is tremendous variation in the ages at which the actual symptoms begin. Orene sometimes sees menopausal patients as young as thirty-seven and as old as fifty-six, so it can be risky to dismiss a woman's anxieties with the simple diagnosis: "You're too young for that."

One of Orene's patients stopped menstruating in her early thirties and could not be made to menstruate or ovulate even with the use of several fertility hormones. She indeed experienced an unusually early menopause. Other patients, still having fairly regular periods at age fifty-five, wonder if they'll ever be finished. Clinically, they must be considered premenopausal.

One fifty-three-year-old patient with fibroid tumors of

the uterus continued to have periodic bleeding, which was not normal menstruation since her hormone levels indicated that she was actually postmenopausal (although she did not remember any menopausal symptoms). Eventually she underwent a hysterectomy to remove the tumors.

There's also an enormous variation in the response of different women's bodies to the changes of menopause. Some seem to breeze through with scarcely a symptom. These are the women who may think it's a matter of attitude, or even of spirituality, which certainly can be part of the picture. But other women, despite their positive approach and leaning on the Lord, do have a difficult time. Physical difficulties during menopause do not mean that someone is weak, self-centered, or unspiritual.

If you find menopause "about as tough as trimming a hangnail," as one patient expressed it, thank God for that. But be sure to listen to your less fortunate friends. Offer your compassion, emotional support, and physical help. Please don't tell them, "It's all in your head"!

Let's see what physically happens to your body during menopause. It's a bit complex, but if you'll bear with us, we think you'll marvel, as we do, at what an immensely complex structure the Lord has created. And if you'll spend a little time learning the interrelationships that bring it all together, you'll have a far clearer understanding of why you feel as you do and of what can be done to help you.

The Normal Reproductive Cycle

This natural cycle is really a most incredible feedback system or chain reaction in which your body prepares itself for a specific event: the fertilization of the ovum and development of the embryo. It all begins when your hypothalamus, a glandular control center in your brain, signals your pituitary gland to release a follicle stimulating hormone (FSH) into your blood stream (see illustration 1).

Inside your ovaries are follicles, little cystic structures or depressions, that contain eggs. When the FSH reaches your ovaries, it stimulates the maturation of one of the many folli-

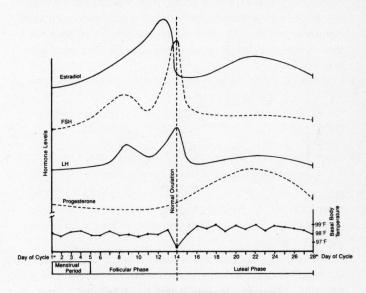

PHYSIOLOGY OF MENSTRUAL CYCLES

Illustration 1

cles (see illustration 2). A thick layer of cells surrounding the developing follicle secretes estrogen in a very specific form called "estradiol." Meanwhile, the increasing estrogen circulates in your blood and acts on your uterus to prepare it for the arrival of the egg. These activities occur during the "estrogen" or "follicular" phase of the menstrual cycle, which lasts about fourteen days (with day number one being the day the menses start).

Now the increasing estrogen in your blood triggers the hypothalamus to stimulate the pituitary gland to increase further the secretion of FSH and to cause a surge of luteinizing hormone (LH) to be released. This surge stimulates the follicle even more and it ruptures. Ovulation occurs. The egg or ovum separates from the follicle and is propelled into your fallopian tubes and into the uterus. The ruptured follicle (the cystic structure that contained the egg) remains on the ovary and becomes the corpus luteum or "yellow body," a yellow cellular structure. The corpus luteum secretes estrogen but, in addition, it releases a second major ovarian hormone, progesterone.

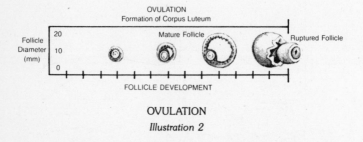

OVULATION

Illustration 2

Progesterone governs the second or lutual phase of the cycle by further developing and maturing the lining of the uterus in preparation for implantation of a fertilized ovum. In other words, the corpus luteum is necessary to complete the preparation of the uterine lining for pregnancy because of the progesterone and estrogen which its cells secrete.

If no pregnancy occurs, the corpus luteum degenerates, and progesterone and estrogen production falls. The endometrium (the lining of the uterus) breaks away from the uterine wall, and you begin to menstruate. With the fall in progesterone and estrogen, your hypothalamus again signals your pituitary to secrete FSH, and your cycle begins again.

It's like a glorious musical round, which progresses from one part to the next, and finally returns to the beginning theme, only to repeat the cycle once again(see illustration 3).

Perimenopause

As you become older, your ovarian function begins to decline and fewer follicles mature and ovulate as they become more resistant to FSH stimulation. Since these follicles secrete estrogen, there is less estrogen and also very much less progesterone flowing through your bloodstream. Your pituitary senses this decline in estrogen and begins to produce more FSH and LH in an effort to stimulate the aging

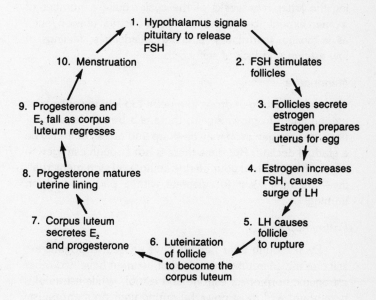

1. Hypothalamus signals pituitary to release FSH

2. FSH stimulates follicles

3. Follicles secrete estrogen Estrogen prepares uterus for egg

4. Estrogen increases FSH, causes surge of LH

5. LH causes follicle to rupture

6. Luteinization of follicle to become the corpus luteum

7. Corpus luteum secretes E_2 and progesterone

8. Progesterone matures uterine lining

9. Progesterone and E_2 fall as corpus luteum regresses

10. Menstruation

THE MENSTRUAL CYCLE

Illustration 3

ovary to ovulate. FSH levels continue to rise, sometimes reaching as much as thirteen times what they formerly were; and the LH levels rise as much as three times.

No wonder your menstrual cycle begins to change! There is a gradual drift from ovulatory cycles to shortened cycles and then to nonovulation. Either the follicle phase or lutual phase shortens, and some women's cycles decrease to twenty-four days or even less. The periods may become irregular, closer together, and finally cease altogether. Without a balance of progesterone, the lining of the uterus may be constantly stimulated by estrogens, and the periods become heavier. All kinds of patterns are possible, depending upon how quickly the ovarian function declines.

Since the ratio of estrogen to progesterone varies during the latter two weeks of the cycle, quite a number of women experience symptoms of premenstrual tension, such as irritability, tearfulness, bloating, headaches, feelings of low esteem and lack of self worth.

Menopause

At last, estrogen drops to a point too low to cause your uterine lining to grow. Again, there is a tremendous variation; the estrogen drop may be sharp and quick, or it may be a gradual decline. But once there is not enough estrogen to trigger the growth of your uterine lining, you stop menstruating. You may want to celebrate with a pad-and-tampon burning!

Postmenopause

Even though your periods have ceased, estrogens are still present. In addition to estradiol, women have two other estrogenic hormones: estrone and estriol. While estradiol is paramount and most powerful during your premenopausal days, estrone is the principle estrogen of the postmenopause.

A fascinating fact about estrone is that it's produced in "extraglandular sites" (outside of the glands) and uses hormone precursors or forerunners secreted by your ovary and adrenal gland. These precursor hormones are the male hormones, androstenedione and testosterone.

In certain tissues, including fat cells, these precursors are converted to estrone by changing only a small part of the structural formula, which means the more fat cells you have, the more estrogen your body is equipped to manufacture. That's good, in terms of menopausal symptoms, and explains why heavy women often have an easier menopause. However, it's bad in terms of cancer risk. Obese postmenopausal women run a four-to-five times greater risk of uterine cancer than their thinner sisters, which is the price they pay for continuing estrogen exposure. Illustration 4 charts your hormone production changes from puberty to menopause. However, the real question should be: "Am I still ovulating?"

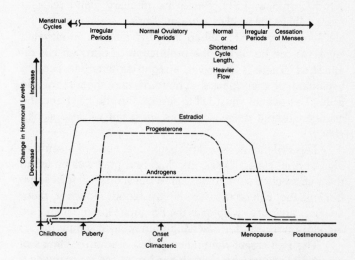

CORRELATION OF MENSTRUAL CYCLE WITH HORMONE
PRODUCTION THROUGHOUT LIFE
Illustration 4

Until recently many women concluded after skipping several cycles that they were no longer ovulating. This sometimes erroneous conclusion has contributed in part to an unplanned pregnancy—the so-called menopausal baby. Thus, while the ovaries are undergoing changes, you may still be ovulating occasionally. The ovaries are producing some estrogens, but the triggering mechanism between the pituitary gland and the ovaries is not enough to induce monthly ovulation. Even with a six-month interlude between periods, the ovaries may still muster enough estrogen to make you ovulate a few more times.

Some people have used the timeline of one year since the last menstrual period to determine whether you're postmenopausal and nonovulating. However, doctors no longer have to make assumptions based on a time limitation. Through a blood test we can do an analysis of the pituitary gland hormone, FSH. Since the pituitary gland releases more FSH as the level of estrogen drops, we measure for the elevation of the FSH. When the FSH reaches an elevated level, we can be certain the production of estrogen has diminished. There is, however, a slight lag-time between the beginning of menopausal symptoms and the rise of the FSH. The ovaries must fail to respond to the FSH and the estrogen output decrease before the FSH will rise significantly.

This FSH analysis will probably cost about the same as your annual gynecological checkup and may well be worth the investment for the unanswered questions it resolves. Estrogens, too, can be measured in the blood. However, these analyses are not as helpful as the FSH measurement and are therefore not used for assessing menopausal symptoms.

The Pap smear maturation index is another means of assessing hormone function. It has been used for many decades, but is not extremely accurate. Taking the maturation index involves scraping the vaginal wall with the Pap stick to obtain vaginal (not cervical) cells. There are three different kinds of vaginal cells: parabasal (small, oval or round cells with a relatively large nucleus), intermediate (large, polygon-shaped cells with a small nucleus), and superficial (also polygon-shaped but with a larger nucleus). In childhood, almost all your cells are parabasal. During that time the maturation index will read something like this: 80 percent parabasal, 20 percent intermediate, 0 percent superficial.

As the reproductive organs mature, the index moves toward the right. Once you have begun ovulation, you have both intermediate cells and superficial cells (for example, 0 percent parabasal, 70 percent intermediate, 30 percent superficial). Thus, you have both estrogen and progesterone components working on those vaginal cells.

During menopause, the maturation index is all intermediate (0 percent parabasal, 100 percent intermediate, 0 percent superficial). Finally, when your system is no longer producing estrogen, you return to a parabasal stage similar to that of your childhood years (100 percent parabasal, 0 percent intermediate, 0 percent superficial). To calculate the maturation index, the technician must read 100 cells and figure the percentage of each cell type. This calculation can be done with the Pap smear as long as an extra slide of the vaginal wall cells is obtained.

These changes in cell types are a good indication of how complicated the changes in a woman's body are. No wonder our metabolism sometimes affects our emotions.

Orene always relies on a blood FSH level before making a final diagnosis about whether a woman is menopausal. A woman who has no hot flashes and has stopped having menstrual periods is a good candidate for an FSH test. So is a woman who experiences the opposite symptoms of having hot flashes but continuing her menstrual periods. In both these instances, the physical symptoms do not completely correlate; therefore a third tool is needed for diagnosis.

Chances are, however, that you will be the first to realize that you're beginning menopause. Your clues will be any of a number of different symptoms, and we'll help you to identify them in the next chapter.

Chapter Three

IS ANYONE ELSE HERE
FEELING WARM?

"How will I know I've reached menopause?" a member of a bridge foursome asked her somewhat older friends.

"You'll know, honey. You'll know!" responded the woman to her right, as she fanned herself with a tally card.

The hot flash, or to be more accurate the hot flush, is probably the most talked-about symptom of menopause. It's generally described as a feverlike sense of growing warmth,which seems to stem from the very core of your being, building until you may feel your chest and face flushing and breaking into perspiration. At night, flushes may take the form of so-called "night sweats," when a woman wakes up drenched and, consequently, sometimes becomes chilled.

Hot flushes or sweats may begin while you are still menstruating fairly regularly. Again, there is infinite variation. Certain women have them only at night. Sometimes, they are just an occasional annoyance, a cause for finding an open window or shedding a sweater. Menopausal women learn to layer their clothes and to avoid long-sleeved wool turtlenecks. Some learn to recognize the onset of a flush and to lessen its impact by shedding or fanning before it peaks. For the more severely affected, hot flushes may come as often as every twenty minutes and feel so intense that, as one woman put it, "I long to jump into a cold shower." They leave these women chilled, exhausted, and embarrassed. The duration of a flush is different for different women. It may last only a few seconds or may persist for several minutes.

Hot flushes occur in seventy-five to eighty percent of

menopausal women, but for fifty percent of those who experience them, they'll cease in a year. For twenty-five to fifty percent, they will last longer than five years. A few women have to tolerate them for eight to ten years. Treatment with hormones may postpone flushes so that symptoms may recur after therapy ceases.

Hot flushes seem to be stimulated by an overly warm environment. Unfortunately, they seldom occur when we could most use them such as, while riding a ski lift or waiting for a bus on a subzero day. They can also be triggered by close body contact with another warm human being, and consumption of hot liquids or alcohol tends to increase the number and severity. Getting flustered over a situation can also bring on a hot flash. A salesclerk told us that anytime she had a minor confrontation with a customer, she'd feel a hot flush beginning. This onset caused her such embarrassment that she couldn't go on with the conversation.

The medical term for the hot flush is "vasomotor instability," meaning that the peripheral or close-to-the-surface blood vessels expand to produce the symptoms. Although a central chemical in the brain is thought to initiate the flush, no one knows exactly what it is. Doctors do know, however, that the hot flush is an effect of decreasing estrogen levels on the hypothalamus, the gland which, among other things, regulates body temperature and the dilatation of these superficial blood vessels.

The flush has also been defined as a thermo-regulatory disorder. Women often wonder if there actually is a measurable rise in body temperature, and the answer is yes. Your fingers, toes, and cheeks do rise in temperature. In fact, the cheek may rise about 0.7 degrees centigrade, the finger temperature somewhat less. The heart rate also increases during the onset of the flash, then slows immediately afterwards. Oral temperatures have registered no increase, but a drop of as much as one degree centigrade occurs after the onset of the flush.

As you can see, we've come a long way from the days when doctors considered the flush a psychological phenomenon, not a physical occurrence, but they are still a very real problem to the woman who is awakened repeatedly during the night.

MENSTRUAL CHANGES

Probably long before you experience a hot flash, if you ever do, you will notice changes in your periods. Orene likes to deal with the entire spectrum of the climacteric, rather than just menopause, because these changes occur considerably before the more classic menopausal symptoms. Premenstrual syndrome (PMS), for instance, while occurring at any age in the menstruating female, is often exaggerated during the climacteric—the peak years from about thirty-six to fifty when the ovaries begin to wind down.

By definition, premenstrual tension occurs before the period and improves afterwards. Typically PMS symptoms begin the week before menstruation, but in some cases as early as two weeks before the period. Research indicates that the symptoms may be precipitated by the change in the ratio of progesterone to estrogen, hormones present during the luteal phase of the cycle, with either too little progesterone or a relatively high amount of estrogen (see illustration 1, ch. 2).

Much has been written about premenstrual tension in the past few years. The subjective nature of many of the symptoms makes it difficult to separate hormone-related symptoms from stress-induced symptoms. Physical symptoms are weight gain from water retention, bloating, headaches, and craving for sweets. Psychological symptoms include irritability, tearfulness, anxiety with mild depression, and loss of feeling of self-worth.

If these symptoms handicap a woman in performing well in the home or on the job, she can and should receive help. However, the great majority of women consider these manifestations a minor bother and come to accept them as a cyclical part of their personalities. In fact, Orene had a patient, an artist who asked to be placed on oral contraceptives, both for birth control and to control her outbursts of temper and mild depression before menstruation. Returning three or four months later, she asked to be taken off the medication and explained, "I've lost all my creativity and ability to paint. I never dreamed that these mood swings were a vital part of being a sensitive, imaginative artist. I'm much better off with my natural cyclic pattern than with the more placid, smooth moods which the pill seems to create."

It is no fluke that most pregnant women experience a last minute surge of energy just before the baby arrives. The change in the hormone ratio in their bodies causes this sensation of energy, which inspires them to tidy the nest in anticipation of the baby's arrival. Although much has been written on the negative aspects of premenstrual tension, perhaps it too is not always a syndrome to be corrected or changed.

PMS symptoms may become more intense as a woman grows closer to menopause. As the ovary begins to fail, doctors often find an "inadequate luteal phase," when the progesterone production from the ovary diminishes. The result is that some women develop spotting before the menstrual flow. (As we saw in chapter 1, the withdrawal of hormones causes the menstrual flow.) This decreased output of progesterone can also intensify premenstrual tension.

During the perimenopause (the beginning of ovarian decline, from age thirty to fifty or so), it is more common to have menstrual abnormalities, such as flooding, clotting, and irregular periods. Physicians become worried when a woman of this age suddenly develops heavy bleeding (defined as requiring more than eight pads in a twenty-four-hour period), too-frequent periods, or bleeding between periods, since it is more common to develop precancer or cancer of the endometrium at this age. Sometimes a dilatation and curettage (a minor surgical procedure which consists of scraping the uterine lining) is indicated, so doctors can determine if an early cancer of the endometrium (the lining of the uterus) or a precancer is present.

Heavy bleeding, of course, can also stem from fibroids, which are usually benign tumors appearing in the muscle layer of the uterus wall. Polyps (benign, fingerlike growths extending from the lining of the uterus) can also produce abnormal bleeding, most often bleeding between periods. When women past the age of menopause continue to bleed periodically, doctors usually recommend a D & C. If this doesn't improve the bleeding pattern, a hysterectomy may be indicated.

SLEEP DISTURBANCES

The irritability of some women in menopause may not be emotional in origin, but physical, since women who are awakened by hot flushes or night sweats are also suffering from sleep deprivation. They may be just plain exhausted.

However, other forms of sleep disturbance may occur in menopause, quite apart from flushes. They've been identified by researchers from electroencephalogram (EEG) readings, which measure brain waves during sleep. Sometimes there is a decrease in the amount of REM (periods of rapid eye movement during which sleep is most restful), which some doctors believe is related to decreased estrogen. Others say that sleep-disordered breathing (when a person actually fails to breathe for an abnormally long period of time) can also result from estrogen deprivation.

You may recall that sleep deprivation is a tool used by some cults to change members' ways of thinking and responding. It's also a favored way to weaken the will and obtain information from prisoners of war. Obviously a woman who is suffering from any one of these sleep disturbances will not be able to cope with daily situations as well as she usually does.

BODY CHANGES

Change in the body is the part of aging no one likes to consider, but it is common for both men and women. For instance, the "gravity factor" causes everything to become a little lower. Women's hips and stomachs enlarge; men's chests are said to "fall," resulting in the familiar pot belly.

Let's look at some of the body changes generally ascribed to menopause.

Breast Change

Perhaps you've heard some women lament that their breasts grew smaller after menopause, while others say just the opposite. There is no uniform change that occurs during or after menopause. Some women do experience a diminution of breast size, related to the estrogen decrease. Others may find they need a larger bra cup size.

While breasts are usually less tender during the premenstrual phase of the cycle, women can still develop a tender nodule. This nodule may remain after their menstrual cycle and could be a benign fibrocystic breast change. However, beware of assuming that a lump is nothing to worry about; in chapter 7, we'll discuss breast malignancies. Certainly women should be aware that the risk that a lump, tender or not, is malignant increases during the postmenopausal years.

Weight Gain

Adding pounds may be an indirect consequence of menopause. Although estrogen declines, androgens (anabolic steroids) are still produced by the ovary; this imbalance may cause an increase in weight. More likely, however, additional pounds are the result of the general slowing down of your metabolism as you grow older. You simply can't eat as much as before without gaining weight. (Do you know you can gain weight in a year by using an electric rather than a manual typewriter?) Do you exercise regularly? Exercise will help you maintain your regular weight. See chapter 7 for some other compelling reasons for exercising.

Facial Hair

Many postmenopausal women are dismayed to find increased growth of facial hair, particularly on the upper lip and chin.

"Am I going to become the bearded lady of the circus?" they ask anxiously. Or worse yet, "Will I become like a man?" It's true that there may be a new fuzziness on your face or an increase in dark hair growth. Sometimes it will be quite coarse. But the growth is limited since it's caused by the change in hormonal balance.

As we've seen, the ovaries produce both male and female hormones. As the ovaries fail and cease producing estrogen, they continue to produce androstendione and testosterone, which convert peripherally to estrone. However, the change in this delicate balance of the relative proportions of male/female hormones can affect the hair follicles and actually increase hair growth. It is not generally a major change and need not be treated with hormones.

Skin Changes

The skin dryness and loss of turgor (puffiness) we see in women of this age are probably due to aging in general. More often, these conditions are caused by exposure to sun (deep tanning) rather than by hormonal changes. You'll note that women who have oily skin tend not to have the wrinkle problems of women with dry skin. However, generalized thinning of the skin related to loss of elasticity does result in wrinkling. The beneficial use of estrogens to retard or prevent wrinkling is just not documented, even though the skin does have estrogen receptors. A skin moisturizer will do much more to keep the skin from wrinkling than any estrogens. If you use sun screen for many years before menopause, you may prevent a good bit of wrinkling.

Headaches

Some women seem to associate headaches with menopause, and certainly we have observed headaches in women within forty-eight to seventy-two hours following an *oophorectomy*, the surgical removal of the ovaries. This onset correlates with the clearance of estrogens from the body and the onset of hot flushes. There is some concern that the woman with migraine headaches may have even worse headaches with estrogen replacement therapy. However in Orene's experience, this is generally not true. In fact, the headaches associated specifically with menopause will often cease if estrogen is given.

Infertility

The ultimate consequence of menopause, of course, is infertility, although, as we noted in the last chapter, it's possible for the ovaries to have a late surge even after some months without a period. This is unusual, but the ovaries *could* produce enough hormones for the follicle to mature and the egg to be released.

For this reason, do not be lulled into a false sense of security. Orene recommends some form of mechanical birth control until *a year after the last menstrual period*. The importance of responsible birth control after age forty cannot be overemphasized.

Orene recently watched the trauma of a forty-two-year-old nurse who found she was pregnant, even though she'd used a diaphragm. She learned from a perinatologist, a specialist in high risk pregnancy and delivery, that the chances of a chromosome deficiency in her baby were one in thirty-nine. The probability of having a perfect baby diminishes and the chance of infant deformities, such as Mongolism, increases with the aging ovum. "To think I've done this when it could have been prevented by sterilization!" the nurse said.

Kerry, another patient, had a fifteen year old daughter but had been unable to conceive again. Orene did some basic infertility testing, including sperm count and measurement of hormones. She found no problem, but Kerry still did not become pregnant.

When she reached forty, they discussed her changing body chemistry and the risk of chromosome abnormality at her age. Amniocentesis, or tapping of the amniotic fluid and growing cells to check for chromosome abnormalities, cannot be performed until about fourteen weeks, and the results do not come back for four more weeks. By then the fetus is over four months old, and the mother can hear the heartbeat and feel the movement of her baby. "I just do not want to face the heart-rending decision of whether to continue with a pregnancy if I know there can't be a healthy, normal child," Kerry realized. Therefore she decided it would be wise to have a sterilization procedure, since a reason for her infertility had never been found and she still had some risk of pregnancy. (It was then that she received news that her daughter, now eighteen and married, would be having a child in seven months. Kerry would get to enjoy a new baby after all.)

For many Christian women abortion is not an option, since they believe interfering with the pregnancy is killing a human being. If you are over forty, we urge you to talk with your husband about what precautions you should take to guard against conception. Perhaps he will feel that a vasectomy is appropriate, or possibly you would feel more comfortable with a tubal sterilization.

The inability to reproduce at the end of the climacteric is truly a wonderful part of God's plan for us. No matter how healthy we may be, we no longer have the same body stamina to carry a fetus for nine months. There are more frequent medical complications and a poorer labor response of the uterus. So it is truly a protective mechanism to have the reproductive capability taken from us in the late forties and early fifties.

Urinary Incontinence

Certain changes in the urinary system seem to be exaggerated during the menopause. These include increasing stress incontinence and a sensation of burning when urinating, which may come with thinning of estrogen-dependent tissues.

When addressing a group on the climacteric, Cynthia Rector, R.N., a member of the staff at the Center for Climacteric Studies in Gainesville, Florida, frequently asks, "Anybody here have trouble with leaking when you laugh?"

"The women all look at each other and nod," she says. "But it's something they tend not to admit to each other, or even to their physicians."

The gynecologist watches for this problem in Caucasian women who have had several children, which may have caused the pelvic diaphragm to weaken, often "drooping" the pelvic organs and bladder. The angle of insertion of the urethra (the canal through which urine is voided) to the bladder is changed. Any pressure exerted by the abdominal muscles, as in lifting, sneezing, or jumping, is relayed to the bladder, which results in a loss of urine.

If the problem is mild, it can be solved by wearing a thin pad when exercising or when a cold causes frequent coughing. A more severe problem might make it necessary to wear a pad daily, whether going out socially or doing housework at home.

Severe stress incontinence, that which is incapacitating and keeps a woman inactive because of fear of embarrassment, should be corrected surgically. The surgical procedure usually involves removal of the uterus and an additional procedure to restore support to the bladder and recreate the urethral-bladder angle to allow proper control of urination.

Incidentally, younger women can have a problem, too. Many college girls who are active in gymnastics have stress incontinence, and we don't really know how to solve it. Jumping on a trampoline or any exercise that requires a lot of bouncing will also produce the difficulty. Likewise women who do aerobic exercising may leak urine when they do jumping jacks.

Vaginal Dryness

Here's another problem women hesitate to talk about. If a doctor notices it and questions her, there's likely to be an "Oh, yes!" outpouring of concern.

The trouble with vaginal dryness is that it's not an early symptom of menopause, but a delayed consequence of the loss of estrogen to the tissues. Women may not realize that it's related to menopause. In fact, a woman may go through an uneventful menopause, without hot flashes or any other particular difficulty, then perhaps a year or two later, find she has a problem because of dryness and actual thinning of the vaginal lining.

One patient said to Orene, "My marriage is better than ever. It's a good time in my life. Yet intercourse is impossible for me." She had no idea that her problem was related to change of life.

Another woman reported that intercourse left her with the pain of an "internal pavement burn." Fortunately, this condition can be reversed, and we'll describe how in the next chapter.

Osteoporosis

Osteoporosis is the thinning and increased porosity or honey-combing of the bones, which occurs naturally with aging. It happens to men and women, but it is greatly accelerated in postmenopausal women, affecting about twenty-five percent after a natural menopause and up to fifty percent after surgical menopause without hormone replacement. Although this process begins early in the climacteric, it may not become obvious for many years.

Moreover, the calcium, which you take in from your diet and from supplements to help rebuild bone is absorbed less and excreted more as you reach menopause. If you are one of the following types, you are prone to this condition: very thin women; those with small bones; white women with fair complexions; Oriental women; women who have never been pregnant; and those whose grandmothers, mothers, or sisters have had osteoporosis.

"Little old ladies" with dowagers' humps are little because they've suffered fractures of their porous, fragile vertebrae. Follow the process with us.

First, one side of a vertebra tilts and begins to curve toward the backbone, producing "wedging." Then the entire vertebra collapses. When several vertebrae collapse, the rib cage tilts down, a hump appears at the top of the back, the spine curves outward, and the abdomen protrudes. A woman can lose two inches of height in a few weeks and as much as eight inches with subsequent fractures!

That's not all. Women with osteoporosis are also prone to fractures of the wrist (the Colles fracture, when both bones of the arm usually slide over the wrist bones) as the result of a fall. However once this fracture is set, it will heal without any lasting effect.

Far more disabling and truly life threatening are older women's hip fractures of the upper part of the femur. Approximately two hundred thousand women over age forty-five fracture their hips each year. Fewer than half of these women regain full function. Hip fractures are the leading cause of accidental death in elderly white women in this country today and the twelfth leading cause of death in America. Fifteen percent die soon after the fracture and thirty percent within a year.

Death stems not from the fracture itself but from three

different conditions resulting from their confinement. First is pneumonia. Second is a rare occurrence called a "fat embolus," in which fatty cells from the bone marrow are found in the blood stream. Third is thrombophlebitis or a blood clot in a leg vein. If a clot breaks off and goes to the lung, forming a pulmonary embolus, it can be fatal. Pinning the hip surgically, if this is possible, to get the patient on her feet again decreases the risk of thrombosis. Elderly people who are immobile also lose bone mass quickly, because they lose the mineral content (such as calcium) of the bone.

Osteoporosis is an extremely serious problem, particularly with today's increased life spans. Fortunately, it can be prevented if you begin early enough. We'll suggest how in chapter 7.

Increased Vascular Disease

In some ways, women are physically superior to men, less prone to high blood pressure and heart disease, *until* they go through menopause. The Framingham study, utilizing 2,873 women over a twenty-four year time span, showed that there is clearly an increased incidence of heart disease immediately after menopause.

High density lipoproteins (HDL) protect our bodies from cardiovascular disease, because they remove excess cholesterol from the cell. Estrogens increase high density lipoprotein levels; and inversely, a decrease in estrogen lowers these levels and increases cholesterol and triglycerides. Postmenopausal women lose their natural protection from cardiovascular disease.

One might think that estrogen replacement therapy would protect women from heart disease—specifically, heart attacks—after menopause. The Framingham study, as well as others, does not support this theory.

A Final Word

Are you feeling a bit overwhelmed by the scope of the body changes during and following menopause? Please don't. Detailed information on coping with these physical changes is just a chapter away.

Remember, too, it's important not to blame every single out-of-the-ordinary feeling you have on menopause or always to assume you're experiencing "just another symptom." Other problems, totally unrelated to menopause, might arise at this time of your life. It's wise to report any symptoms promptly to your physician and to be sure to have regular checkups.

We've mentioned a number of menopausal symptoms which aren't always welcome. The good news is that there are also some positive changes!

First, fibroids, those usually benign but sometimes troublesome tumors of the uterus, regress after menopause. Once the hormone stimulation is gone, fibroids usually diminish in a year or so, a situation which will be noticeable to your physician in a pelvic exam.

Also, endometriosis diminishes. Endometriosis is a benign condition where the glandular tissue that lines the uterus is found within the abdomen (for unknown reasons), located as tiny implants *on* the ovaries, uterus, and connecting ligaments. Endometriosis can produce symptoms such as pain, painful intercourse, and heavy menstrual periods, plus infertility. After menopause, the pain may diminish and, of course, the periods will stop.

Never forget the obvious benefit of menopause—no more periods. No more cramps or chills. No more planning ahead with one eye on the calendar. No more pads or tampons. No more PMS or monthly mood swings. You are finally free from the discomforts and inconveniences of menstruation!

Chapter Four

COPING WITH THE CHANGES

It has been a long, hard night in the labor room for Orene's patient, Kim, and her husband, Jeff. Orene has participated in their discouragement, the questioning of why Kim's labor is so long, the fears that all may not be right. Everyone is tired, and suddenly, it's time to move to the delivery room.

Kim is very uncomfortable. She's been taught in Lamaze classes how to push, but at times she's sure she didn't learn well enough. Now she wonders if she can push one more time.

Orene encourages her, "Yes, you can!"

The baby's heartbeat, which is monitored carefully, drops. Orene tells Jeff she may have to use forceps.

"Forceps!" he cries, as though this would be the end of the world.

Orene encourages Kim to push again, with her very hardest effort, and at last the baby's head begins moving out of the birth canal.

Everything happens at once. Orene makes the episiotomy, and the baby's glistening head emerges. At this point it's extremely important to deliver the shoulders and the rest of the baby, because the infant can't breathe and the cord is usually not providing any respiratory benefits. Very quickly, the shoulders are delivered. The baby, a good-sized boy, is quiet. Orene places him on the mother's abdomen as she suctions his tiny mouth. At last, he cries and a tremendous sense of relief spreads through the entire delivery room, from the husband to the patient to Orene and the nurses.

What a sound of beauty is that lusty yowl! What perfection is that slippery little body, from the still slightly flattened features of the ruddy face to the tiny fingers and toes! To hear that lusty cry, to hold a perfectly formed newborn is one of life's greatest privileges. No matter if it's the first or the thousand-and-first time, an obstetrician-gynecologist marvels that our bodies can produce such a beautiful new creation.

As an obstetrician, Orene knows that a new life is so complex, and *we* are limited in what we can do to form it. That the factors to create a new life come together so perfectly is truly a miracle of the Lord.

Once you were that wonderful baby. Once you may have been that mother. Now you have reached the time of the climacteric, but you are still God's beautiful creation. The wonder is that the body functions so well, despite the many changes. Actually these changes can be extremely positive when you understand what's happening to you and when you're aware of the vast spectrum of coping mechanisms which are open to you. Many women, of course, cope very nicely on their own, but there's no reason today for anyone to resign herself to suffering silently or to feel she must simply act tough.

Your Role in Coping

You've already taken the first step in coping by reading this book. You're exploring, educating yourself as to what to expect. Forearmed with knowledge, you can deal with irrational fears or "old tapes" passed down by mothers or grandmothers, so they don't cloud your anticipation of what can be an extremely satisfying passage in your life.

Your next step, if you have any questions or problems, is to see your doctor. If you have an uneventful climacteric, and/or you are well satisfied with your internist or your GP, he or she may be the perfect person to guide you through this time. If you've established a comfortable rapport with your obstetrician through the years, consult with him or her.

However if you have special needs at this time, don't be

embarrassed about shopping for a new doctor. It's extremely important to find someone with whom you can communicate effectively. You needn't settle for a "Yes doctor" relationship. Fortunately, there are few physicians today who will simply pat you on the head and tell you to take your estrogen. But if yours does, remember that you have every right to demand education with your treatment. Begin asking other women about their doctors. Call your local medical society. Then speak to a prospective doctor's nurse about your needs. Her response is often a good barometer of the climate of the practice.

When you do see a doctor, have your questions clearly in mind. Most physicians welcome a patient who brings a list of things to ask (provided it isn't several pages long), and they prefer this forethought to repeated telephone calls of "I forgot's." Nevertheless, doctors also appreciate your being sensitive and not demanding more than is reasonable. It's helpful, too, if you can be aware of a backlog of waiting patients. You might say, "I know you're running behind, but I wish you could find time to give me a little more help." This request gives your physician the option of responding now or possibly phoning you at another time.

Another tip: if your doctor hasn't answered all your questions on a particular day, make sure the nurse is aware of your needs. She may be able to help you, or she will ask the doctor to call you. You are paying for services, and there's no reason for you to go home feeling that you're not being cared for.

Whatever you do, don't decide to alter your treatment or medication on your own, without checking with your doctor, and, if you are seeing more than one specialist, be sure each is aware of the medications you take.

Your Doctor's Role

Let's examine some of the tools that your physician may suggest for coping with physical symptoms. Because estrogen replacement is such a complex topic, and because Orene has found it's necessary only for twenty to twenty-five percent of all women, we'll cover the use of estrogen in the next chapter. Let's look first at the options that are available for coping with specific symptoms.

NONESTROGEN TREATMENTS

Exaggerated PMS Symptoms

As we mentioned in the last chapter, sometimes women who suffer from premenstrual syndrome find their symptoms exaggerated as the ovaries begin to fail. These symptoms are not a part of menopause, but a facet of that broader transition period, the climacteric.

Treatment is not well defined, because the syndrome's hormonal causes and effects are unclear, although a great deal of research is currently being done in this area. The various approaches usually depend on the severity of symptoms. For instance, women with mild cyclic changes may benefit from vitamin B_6 and/or the diuretic spironolactone. More severe symptoms of the premenstrual syndrome may require the use of hormonal therapy. Synthetic progesterone (the progestins) is not helpful in treating the symptoms. Pure progesterone (a synthetically prepared steroid that contains the same molecular structure as the progesterone the body makes) has been found to be quite effective when given a week to ten days before the menstrual period.

However, there are several problems with this therapy. First, oral progesterone is not absorbed by the body, so the drug must be administered by injection or as a suppository. Second, the Federal Food and Drug Administration (FDA) has yet to approve this drug in such high doses as recommended: 200-400 milligram suppositories, one to two times daily in the vagina or rectum. Studies are currently being done that will allow the FDA to approve this therapy.

Sometimes an antidepressant is indicated. However,

you need one that starts working rapidly, and most antidepressants take several weeks to reach a level that gives relief. Some doctors find that an antidepressant called Ascendin is effective in about forty-eight hours, although it is not specifically indicated in the literature for PMS. Beware of tranquilizers during this period. Although your anxiety and irritability are high, you may also feel depressed, an emotional state which tranquilizers might simply intensify.

A low salt diet also has been advocated for women who gain four or five pounds or more (some gain as much as ten) before their periods due to water retention.

Some doctors recommend a dosage of vitamin B_6, 100 to 500 milligrams a day *every* day, not just during the days when PMS exists. The way that vitamin B improves premenstrual tension is not known, but this dosage is well above the recommended daily allowance. This treatment may be continued for six months or long-term, depending upon its effectiveness.

Spironolactone, a diuretic, can also be administered as a long-term medication without side effects. It does not deplete potassium, as many diuretics do, so it does not produce weakness and fatigue. Spironolactone is especially helpful when the PMS includes water retention and should be used only during the days when symptoms are present.

Hot Flashes

Although estrogen replacement therapy is the standard method of treating hot flashes, not all women are candidates for estrogen treatment. Alternatives include biofeedback, progesterone therapy, and such symptom-treating drugs as Bellergal and Cimetidine.

Some women have taught themselves to recognize the onset of a hot flash and can "control it with the mind," as one woman said. The Center for Climacteric Studies in Gainesville, Florida, notes some success in controlling hot flashes by teaching women biofeedback. However, this method is not effective for night sweats since they begin when a woman is asleep and unable to exercise control.

Progesterone, administered either orally as Provera or intramuscularly as Depo-provera will improve hot flashes. But it can cause breakthrough bleeding and spotting; therefore it is not ideal for women who still have a uterus.

However, progesterone is a possible alternative for the woman who has had breast cancer or a surgical menopause. One of Orene's patients who had a radical mastectomy five years ago is now menopausal and having severe hot flashes. What can she use? It's risky to give estrogens because estrogen may stimulate a viable cancer cell. Orene prescribed progesterone since this hormone does not seem to stimulate breast cancer cells as estrogens do. The usual dose of intramuscular progesterone, Depo-provera, is 200 milligrams a month. Oral progestins, such as Provera, are taken daily.

Sometimes a physician treats hot flashes by prescribing nonhormonal medications, which affect the nervous system. Phenobarbitol is an old-fashioned drug given for years by physicians, but it is habitforming and must be used with extreme care. Bellergal, a combination of phenobarbital, ergotrate, and a derivative of belladonna, is more commonly used today. Again, the drug Bellergal could be habitforming, and it should not be used by persons with heart disease or hypertension. As the patient, you should be aware that these drugs treat the symptoms rather than the endocrine cause of the hormone imbalance.

Clonidine (another drug that is effective on the autonomic nervous system and is used to control hypertension) has been reported to be effective in alleviating hot flashes. One research project, however, suggests that it is no better than a placebo, which was also used in the study.

There's been considerable talk about the role of vitamin E in lessening hot flashes, but we do not know of any control studies that confirm its effectiveness. Further, excess doses of vitamin E can lead to blood clots and elevated blood pressure.

Urinary Incontinence

If you have a problem with urinary incontinence, please don't be reticent about discussing it with your doctor. Help is likely to be available.

In the last chapter, we described how stress incontinence is caused by a change in bladder support, which alters the angle between the urethra and the bladder. This change creates a pressure gradient phenomenon, resulting in leakage of urine, particularly when abdominal pressure occurs, as in straining, laughing, coughing, or jumping.

Sometimes Kegel exercises can be used to strengthen the pelvic diaphragm and prevent loss of urine. This exercise involves the voluntary muscle that is used in stopping urination, a muscle called the *pubococcygeus*. With the knees apart, you simply contract and relax the muscle repeatedly, approximately fifteen times, three times a day. Once they know the muscle exists, many women can easily contract it just by imagining they are stopping urination. If you can't, try contracting the muscle when you are urinating, interrupting the flow. Contract, relax. Contract, relax. After you've tried it a few times, you'll be able to do it wherever you are, whether you're cleaning, cooking, driving your car, or sitting at your desk. It's an exercise which is also used in prepared childbirth classes to strengthen the birth canal. Further, it can improve your sex life, as you'll see in chapter 6. Unfortunately, however, the Kegel exercise is not always a totally successful solution for urinary incontinence.

Another treatment is surgical, either through a vaginal approach or an abdominal approach to try to restore the angle between the bladder and urethra. This procedure is usually accompanied by a hysterectomy because the uterus tends to tug on the tissue and to promote loss of support.

Unless there are also frequent urinary tract infections, a repair of this sort is an elective procedure. It's something you must make a decision about yourself. If you are unable to exercise at all, you may want to have it done, but you need to realize that this surgery is not always one-hundred percent successful.

The insertion of a pessary is still another treatment. A pessary is a rubber ring, similar to a diaphragm, except that it is open, without a cup, and quite rigid. It is placed in the vagina and pushes the relaxed bladder and uterus back into a fairly normal position. Usually it is inserted by the gynecologist and can be removed, sterilized, and reinserted every six weeks or so in the office. Some patients learn to replace their own pessaries, thus allowing them the freedom to use them intermittently. For women who are sexually active, knowing how to insert and remove the pessary is important since intercourse is impossible with the pessary in place. Insertion/removal also prevents a chronic inflammation with discharge, which occurs in many continuous users.

Loss of bladder control can also be caused by neurological problems, an inflammation of the urethra, or a vescico-vaginal fistula (a small hole in the bladder which allows it to drain into the vagina). So again, don't assume you know the answers. By all means, see your physician.

Vaginal Dryness, Atrophy

Vaginal estrogen creams are extremely effective in relieving this condition, as we will see in the next chapter. But since blood concentrations of estrogen rise after using estrogen creams, this may not be desirable for everyone. What are the alternatives?

Some women find liberal use of a lubricating jelly, such as K-Y, helpful, both before intercourse and as a nightly application. Some like such preparations as Maxilube or Transilube. Others find A & D ointment more soothing. Beware, however, of Vaseline, for it may be irritating to the tissues.

Also, the "use it or lose it" adage appears to be true. Regular intercourse seems to keep the tissues pliable and to help prevent the narrowing and shortening of the vagina, which can occur with loss of estrogen.

Postmenopausal Bleeding

Any postmenopausal bleeding (other than the artificial "period" which follows the cycle of estrogen-progesterone therapy), is not normal. If you've not had a true period in a year and you bleed unexpectedly, see your doctor. If you have *any* amount of bleeding, from spotting to heavy flow, an office biopsy definitely should be done. If this unscheduled bleeding continues, most physicians feel it's mandatory to do a D & C. An endometrial biopsy is only eighty percent accurate, because it examines only one small piece of tissue, rather than sampling the entire uterine cavity.

Facial Hair

If you're concerned about increased facial hair, several things can be done. First, you can bleach the hair so it is less noticeable. If you want to remove it, a cosmetologist can apply warm wax, which takes the hair off below the skin surface. Of course, you can also use depilatories (creams or liquids, which chemically remove the hair) or shave the hair, but shaving eventually will make the hair feel bristly. Tweezing also works, but it can lead to infection.

Electrolysis, which should be done by a registered electrologist, is the only method that removes hair permanently. However, it takes a long time since each hair must be removed individually with a needle. It is also comparatively expensive, somewhat uncomfortable, and may require many treatments. You should be aware that it won't necessarily leave you completely hair-free forever, because new follicles can produce additional hair.

Remember, there is *no* acceptable hormone treatment available to lessen hair growth during the menopausal years.

Spironolactone and sometimes Prednisone, in special instances, have been used for younger patients but have not
been recommended in the postmenopausal years.

Special Foods and Supplements

Certain nutritionists have advocated certain foods and
food supplements for the menopausal woman. Some suggest attention to potassium intake. Others believe that the
stress of menopause increases nutritional needs for protein,
vitamin C and E, and the B complex. Some nutritionists say
that vitamin A helps to keep mucous membranes moist; they
suggest this vitamin, if it is deficient in the diet, to help alleviate vaginal dryness. Certain herbs such as ginseng, sarsapa-
rilla, and licorice are said to be helpful. However, there's no
scientific indication that any particular foods or supplements
are of benefit for the relief of specific symptoms of menopause. Even vitamin B_6, which seems to bring improvement
to PMS patients, has not at this point been shown to be effective for menopausal women.

In preventing osteoporosis, however, calcium is an essential, and we'll consider that in more detail in chapter 6.

The key to middle-year wellness remains a varied diet
balanced with foods from the four major food groups: cere-
als/grains, fruits/vegetables, dairy products, meat/fish/
fowl.

There was a time, not so very long ago, when many
doctors said to the suffering woman, "You'll just have to
learn to live with it." Those were indeed the dark ages. Be
grateful you're reaching menopause today, when doctors
understand why you feel as you do and are trying to relieve
your physical symptoms. If you and your doctor work together, you can cope with the physical changes that accompany menopause.

Chapter Five

IS ESTROGEN FOR YOU?

"I've noticed that I'm developing a lot of wrinkles and my eyelids are drooping," a smartly dressed patient with dramatic salt-and-pepper hair recently told Orene. "I was thinking about going to a plastic surgeon. But my husband suggested that it would cost a lot less to come to you and get some hormones."

Indeed, some people think that hormone therapy will reverse the aging process and keep them young and feminine forever.

Others, despite acute physical symptoms of menopause, are terrified of the possible increased risk of cancer with estrogen therapy. "Oh, no!" they tell Orene. "I don't want to take that risk. As long as I can keep from going on estrogens, I don't want them."

Neither is accurate in her expectations. Like so many women, they're confused about estrogen replacement therapy, its safety, and what it can and cannot do for them.

Let's examine its advantages and disadvantages. We don't want to leave any of you wishing for more information, so we'll delve into rather technical material in certain instances. Some of it may pertain to you, and some may not. But if you want to find out whether or not estrogen replacement is for you, we urge you to zero in on that which is applicable to you. If you'd like to be helpful to other women who are wondering about estrogen, familiarize yourself with the remainder of the material, too, and use it as a reference when questions arise.

WHAT ESTROGEN CAN AND CANNOT DO

There is no question that estrogen replacement will alleviate hot flashes and night sweats. In fact, Orene's severely afflicted patients call it a miracle drug, for the quick relief it brings. Estrogen also eases some forms of sleep disturbance and headaches, as well as vaginal dryness. It may bring some improvement in incontinence or leakage of urine because it helps restore blood flow to stretched tissue. Estrogen replacement will help prevent osteoporosis or brittle bone disease and, possibly, vascular disease.

However, it is not a successful treatment for other problems. Estrogen will *not* prevent wrinkling of the skin, which is a factor of aging, caused by thinning of the skin and loss of elasticity. Although the presence of estrogen receptors on the skin suggest that there could be some benefit in using estrogen *on* the skin, evidence is not yet conclusive. Also, estrogen will not prevent body changes nor will it reverse stretched and damaged ligaments in the rectal and vaginal areas.

Risks of Estrogen Therapy

The main question women ask about hormone replacement is, "Can it cause cancer?"

If you're talking about breast cancer, the answer depends on which study you read. In 1980, the *Journal of the American Medical Association* reported an increased risk of breast cancer (2.5 times over the general population) in women using 1.25 milligrams of Premarin per day over a three-year period. The risk, however, on .625 milligrams was lower than in the general population, meaning there was no increase in breast cancer on this lower dose. Gambrell, a well-known endocrinologist, reported in 1983 that estrogen therapy does not increase the risk of breast cancer, especially if used with progesterone at the end of each monthly cycle. In general, the danger seems to be small. Patients who had preexisting benign breast disease and received estrogen, however, had a higher rate of breast cancer.

The risk of endometrial cancer is a different story. The danger can be far greater for women who take estrogen. In years past, when long-term and perhaps higher doses of estrogen were given, we saw a resulting increase in cancer of the endometrium, the lining of the uterus. Even today, there is general agreement that the relationship between postmenopausal estrogen intake and the increasing relative risk of developing endometrial cancer is real. In fact, women using estrogens are four to eight times more likely to develop cancer than the general population. However, a three-to-four year treatment is required before a connection between estrogen use and endometrial cancer can be demonstrated. Some doctors have tried to lessen the dosage by prescribing estrogen cyclically (twenty-one days per month), rather than every day, but this effort doesn't seem to protect the patient from endometrial cancer.

Adding a progestin for ten to fourteen days of the cycle, however, is protective. In fact, this hormone can even reverse the precancers (or hyperplasias), which are sometimes found on the lining of the uterus.

Fortunately, the cancers associated with estrogen use seem to have less malignant potential for rapid growth and spread. These are called "well-differentiated" tumors, named to describe what the cells look like microscopically. Thus cancer associated with long-term estrogen use has a high rate of cure.

Some doctors question whether these tumors would have developed anyway, but were diagnosed earlier because a woman on estrogen is watched carefully. At any rate, these Stage I or early cancers have a ninety-five percent, five-year cure rate. However, you should not discount this four-to eight-fold increase in incidence of uterine cancer.

Doctors usually give the lowest effective dose of estrogens when they start a treatment plan. The amount is often .625 milligrams of conjugated estrogen (Premarin) or estrone (Ogen) per day, from day one to day twenty-five. In addition, adding progesterone (Provera, Norlutate, or Aygestin) for the last ten to fourteen days of the cycle (days sixteen to twenty-five) is important for women who still have the uterus. The good news is that progesterone reduces the risk of precancer to zero, and thus should significantly reduce the risk of cancer of the uterus. (A few women use estrogen five out of seven days, rather than stopping for one week. This dosage should still be combined with a progesterone at the end of the month.)

Progesterone can reduce hot flashes and some patients also feel generally better the week progesterone is added to the estrogen. However, there are some negatives to giving progesterone. Fluid retention and, sometimes, breast tenderness may increase. The other negative (and some women really object to this) is that many will experience a menstrual-like period each month after the progesterone is withdrawn. In a sense, that's good, because it means the endometrium is sloughing off cells and effectively decreasing the risk of precancer (hyperplasia), but one of the plusses of going through menopause is not having a period. Weigh these negatives against the benefits of taking hormones.

Occasionally, women who take estrogen and progesterone experience bleeding during the cycle, and doctors dare not assume hormones are the cause. They usually do an endometrial biopsy or a dilatation and curettage (D & C) to be sure the uterus is all right.

Finally, estrogen does not seem to harm diabetics. Unlike oral contraceptives, which affect carbohydrate metabolism (the body's ability to handle glucose intake), estrogen has not been demonstrated to increase blood sugar. If there is a slight change, it isn't enough to cause diabetes or to aggravate the disease in a diabetic.

Screening Before Beginning Hormones

Before you begin hormone therapy, it's important that you have a mammogram, so that you have a baseline against which any breast changes can be noted in succeeding years. (Actually, every menopausal woman should have one, but it is particularly important for those on estrogen.) You should also have an endometrial biopsy if you have any postmenopausal bleeding or if you plan to take estrogen only, without the progesterone. The biopsy tells what the lining of the uterus is like and whether or not there is cancer or precancer already present. If you take estrogen-progesterone, a biopsy should also be performed after two years of treatment or anytime unscheduled vaginal bleeding occurs.

Sometimes doctors see *atypical* adenomatous hyperplasia (a precancer that directly precedes cancer) when they examine the cells under a microscope. This precancer may develop into cancer in the pattern seen in illustration 1. Some doctors would recommend hysterectomy. Others would avoid estrogen therapy and use progesterone for six months, either continuously or possibly for ten days each month. Then they'd check to see if the hyperplasia reverses. This approach should only be done with extreme caution and with a rebiopsy in four to six months.

Pathologists worry about atypical hyperplasia because it can develop into cancer of the uterus. Although, precancer cannot spread, once the cells become cancerous, they can metastasize or spread. Estrogen should not be used if you have atypical adenomatous hyperplasia unless the uterus is removed.

Forms of Estrogen

Estrogen may be given in a number of different forms. Conjugated equine estrogens (such as Premarin, a combination of estrogens from the urine of pregnant mares) are the most frequently used for menopausal symptoms. These are readily absorbed orally. Their effectiveness peaks in three to five hours, and they become ineffective about forty-eight to seventy-two hours after intake.

How much estrogen is necessary to show a change in tests which measure estrogen? The minimal dose that will decrease FSH is .3 milligrams per day; .625 is required to alter vaginal cells in the maturation index of your cycle (see chapter 1).

Estrone, or Ogen, is also a conjugated estrogen but is made of only one estrogen, estrone. It has very little advantage over Premarin and the potency is similar. It also is very effectively absorbed by mouth as well as vaginally. Some patients may have more breast tenderness or water retention with one form and may choose the other to try to reduce minor side effects.

Additional oral estrogen preparations are micronized estradiol (Estrace), ethinyl estradiol (Estinyl) and diethylstilbesterol (DES).

Oral estrogen is usually taken from day one of the month (perhaps starting May 1) through day twenty-five (May 25). You add the progesterone on day sixteen and take both drugs until day twenty-five. Then you take nothing until June 1. If it's done according to a calendar schedule, patients remember to take the hormone better than if they make up their own schedule of certain days on and off.

For a long time, physicians used a preparation that combined estrogen and testosterone. But the testosterone occasionally had some male side effects, and this treatment seems to be out of style today, except under very special circumstances.

There is also an intramuscular form of estrogen, estradiol valerate (Delestrogen), which can be given as an injection every three to four weeks. In a dosage of twenty milligrams, it is as effective as the oral estrogens. Delestrogen is usually reserved for those patients who do not tolerate the oral form well and for a few patients who need high oral doses to bring the FSH levels down and effectively decrease menopausal symptoms.

Other forms of estrogens include a subdermal pellet, which is implanted under the skin in the tissue of the abdominal wall, and a special ring inserted in the vagina. Both allow slow absorption of the estrogen and have the advantage of allowing administration at six-month intervals. However, they are still experimental and are not available until approved by the FDA.

Estrogen creams are extremely effective in treating atrophic vaginitis, an inflammation of the vagina that causes discomfort (either in the vagina itself or sometimes near the introitus or vulva) and can lead to painful intercourse. Sometimes it causes inflammatory discharge and rarely, in extreme cases, postmenopausal bleeding. For most women, the symptoms respond quickly to estrogen creams. Occasionally, however, creams don't reverse the symptoms, and oral estrogens are necessary.

Several brands of creams are on the market. Usually one-half to one full applicator of cream several times weekly is adequate. If you have a significant amount of vaginal atrophy, your doctor may suggest daily or every-other-day application for several weeks, then decreasing the dose to twice weekly. Absorption of one-half applicator of vaginal cream, if used daily, brings the amount of estrogen in the bloodstream to a level equal to using .625 milligrams of Premarin orally per day.

Sometimes a woman's hot flashes may also improve because of the absorption of these dosages into her peripheral blood. However, the woman who cannot take estrogens orally should not use the vaginal cream. If a woman uses the cream for vaginal thinning and dryness only, the dosage can be modified to only several times weekly, thus decreasing blood levels. Some women, once symptoms cease, stop the cream altogether until symptoms arise again.

The bottom line is: Should you take hormones?

The majority of Orene's patients do not. Indeed, some doctors feel that only twenty to twenty-five percent need this pharmaceutical intervention. Make no mistake, hormones are powerful drugs. Hormone replacement is indicated only if you have severe symptoms, such as hot flashes or a dry or atrophic vagina (where intercourse is painful) or if you are at extremely high risk for osteoporosis. The American College of Obstetricians and Gynecologists' technical bulletin states that other uses of estrogen should be approached with caution until further research establishes beneficial effects.

How Much Estrogen Is Enough?

The best dosage of estrogen is the lowest amount that controls the symptoms. It's usually wise to start with .625 milligrams a day and see how that works. If the patient does well on this (has a few hot flashes but they are not incapacitating), this dosage can be continued. If the hot flashes are severe or there are headaches or some emotional difficulties, .9 milligrams per day, and possibly even 1.25, can be tried.

Suppose you are taking 1.25 milligrams and still have severe symptoms. Then your doctor will probably run an FSH test. If the FSH is markedly elevated, two alternatives can be considered. One is to increase the dosage to 2.5 milligrams, which is fairly high. Another is to change to an intramuscular estrogen, which will help the few women who do not absorb oral estrogen well. Of the patients Orene has on estrogen, probably only four or five use the intramuscular injection. They may begin on 20 milligrams of Delestrogen once a month, and often do very well. You might think that the absorption from a monthly injection would not be reliable from day to day, but these patients do not report fluctuations. They say, "I feel so much better on this medication!" The disadvantage to injections, of course, is the coming in for a treatment every month.

How Long Should I Take Estrogen?

The duration of estrogen therapy depends upon your reason for taking this hormone. For hot flushes, you might take estrogen only for twelve to eighteen months, with a progressive reduction in dosage.

Some women who take estrogens for menopausal symptoms wonder, "If I continue to take estrogen, does this mean I won't go through menopause?" In other words, do symptoms begin again when a woman stops hormones?

Yes, most women go through a period of hot flashes after estrogen therapy, no matter how old they are. Sometimes it is necessary to wean a patient from the drug, either by dropping the dose gradually or by starting and stopping until the symptoms are bearable. Atrophic vaginitis is different. Symptoms gradually recur after stopping hormones and never lessen. Thus, this symptom usually requires an indefinite period of therapy, especially in sexually active women.

Prevention of osteoporosis, which we'll discuss at length in chapter 7, is thought to require at least five years of therapy and perhaps longer, but the studies are not complete.

For some women, however, estrogen is not an option.

Who Should Not Take Estrogen?

Estrogen replacement therapy should be avoided if you have had acute liver disease, chronic impaired liver function, breast cancer, or endometrial cancer.

Women with fibrocystic breast disease often wonder if they can take estrogen. It is all right to start estrogens; however, if increased breast tenderness occurs or a new lump appears, your doctor may discontinue therapy or do a mammogram. If there is no increase in breast symptoms, estrogen can be continued, as long as you have careful, periodic breast exams.

Estrogens may not always be advisable for patients with

uterine fibroids, endometriosis, migraines, seizure disorders, familial hyperlipidemia, chronic hypertension, chronic thrombophlebitis, or gallbladder disease.

Fibroids, which are muscle tumors found in the muscular wall of the uterus, are sometimes sensitive to estrogens, and thus can theoretically enlarge with estrogen replacement therapy. They are rarely malignant (only one out of one thousand), and estrogens do not cause them to be malignant. If you know you have fibroids, be sure you have a careful examination of the uterus before beginning estrogen therapy.

Another benign disease, endometriosis (characterized by small glandular implants along the inner lining of the abdominal wall, the ovaries, fallopian tubes, or the ligaments attached to these organs) is sometimes sensitive to estrogens. If you have endometriosis and pelvic pain recurs when you take estrogens, it may be an estrogen effect. Obviously, you should consult your doctor immediately.

Migraines and seizure disorders are not absolute medical contraindications to estrogen replacement therapy. But in some patients they are found more frequently in the premenstrual phase of the menstrual cycle, and therefore are in some way associated with hormones. Since the exact hormonal mechanism or interaction is not known, these women need to be followed more closely when instituting estrogens. In actuality, however, it is rare to have an increase in migraines and seizures with estrogen therapy, in contrast to oral contraceptives, which tend to be more of a problem.

Hyperlipidemia is characterized by elevated cholesterol, triglycerides, and low-density lipoproteins, all associated with greater risk of heart attack. Any woman who has hyperlipidemia must be careful not to increase these lipids, and studies show that some synthetic progestins do just this. However, other studies actually show an increase in the "good" lipids, the *high* density lipoproteins. "Proceed with caution" seems to be the message here.

Chronic hypertension or high blood pressure may rarely become worse when a woman takes estrogens. A person with chronic hypertension might get further elevation of the blood pressure and thus be susceptible to vessel disease, including stroke. Incidences of stroke and thrombophlebitis have not been reported as increased among estrogen users; however, use of estrogen in women with these problems is still controversial. Some studies demonstrate increasing coagulation factors, which would mean women with a history of stroke, heart attack, or prior thrombophlebitis could be at higher risk with estrogen use. However, problems do not occur as frequently as with oral contraceptives, and if they do, the conditions reverse when estrogens are stopped.

Gallbladder disease occurs 2.5 times more frequently in women on estrogens than in the general population. The mechanism is not yet explained, but it most likely has to do with stone-producing bile changes.

All of these conditions must be taken into consideration when choosing estrogen replacement. If you have one of them, it doesn't mean you absolutely cannot take estrogen, but that you may require more frequent observation by your doctor in the early stages of estrogen replacement therapy.

Even when estrogen therapy is not recommended, there can be exceptions, if you work closely with your gynecologist and internist. One of Orene's patients has had an angioplasty and suffers from severe cardiovascular disease, plus a prior episode of phlebitis. Estrogen is generally considered risky in such a case, but she was afflicted with intractable hot flashes and couldn't go a day without being miserable. Now she is on .625 milligrams of estrogen per day and is doing fine. But of course she is monitored very closely, and she understands there may be an increased risk involved in using estrogens. Sometimes, then, women who have conditions that put them at risk can go ahead and take estrogen without feeling like walking time bombs.

We are living in a time when patients enter into the decision-making process. The role of the physician is to educate you and give you your alternatives, then *you* make the decision. You have the choice to start or to stop estrogen therapy. It is not an all-or-nothing matter. You can try estrogen therapy to see how you feel, and you can always stop.

If you do receive hormone therapy, you should plan to see your physician at six- to twelve-month intervals so that your blood pressure can be taken, a breast and pelvic examination performed, and the effectiveness of your treatment evaluated.

Again, we want to emphasize that any postmenopausal bleeding, other than the period that follows the cycle of estrogen-progesterone therapy, is not normal. So if you've not had a true period in a year and you bleed unexpectedly, see your doctor. Any amount of bleeding, from spotting to heavy flow is extremely important to check to determine if cancer or precancer cells are present.

We hope we've shown you that though estrogen replacement can be a godsend for the woman who is truly suffering, it is a powerful drug, which probably only twenty to twenty-five percent of menopausal women actually need.

While Orene never suggests that patients just "grin and bear it," some of us can be too quick to reach for medications. Perhaps our tendency to be such comfort-seekers stems from the flood of commercials today that promise "quick relief" for everything from headaches to hemorrhoids.

Only you can decide how severe your symptoms are. You may be like Evelyn, who elected not to use estrogen for her hot flashes, stating simply, "I decided to sweat it out. After all, this too will pass." Or you may join Martha in hailing estrogen as "a salvation which allows me to sleep and function and feel like a human being again."

Chapter Six

WHAT ABOUT MY SEX LIFE?

"It is widely believed that a postmenopausal woman loses her ability to respond sexually. Of course, this is nothing more than a great cultural fallacy," wrote Dr. William H. Masters, coauthor with Virginia Johnson of *Human Sexual Response* and *Human Sexual Inadequacy.*[1]

Orene's practice corroborates Masters' view. The majority of her counseling for sexual problems is not with women in their fifties, but with those in their twenties and thirties (the very group some of us consider so "liberated" and secure). With few exceptions, difficulty in sexual relationships is not a preoccupation with menopausal women.

Is this because they no longer care? Not at all. In fact, many express that postmenopause is a time of renewal. It is generally not a matter of increased frequency of intercourse, but of new contentment and freedom.

Some women speak of a sense of restoration. It's common to hear, "It's like when we were first married, but better, because we know what pleases each other." Or, "You know how sex is always better when you're away together on vacation? Well, now that the kids are gone, it's like being on vacation all the time." There is a depth of caring and understanding that comes with laughing and crying together for so many years. Now there's time to express that love.

In fact, the menopausal years can be a time of great liberation for couples who have felt inhibited both by the presence of children in the house and by fear of unwanted pregnancy. Now, at last, you needn't wonder if your offspring will hear you, or worse yet, barge in on you. And the freedom of "anyplace, anytime" is freedom indeed. You can be spontaneous, without worrying about pregnancy or the nuisance of birth control.

Once the children are gone, there is more time for each other, plus a deepening of your relationship with your loved one. You can find a new sensitivity and joy in expressing that caring, which results in a contentment that seems fuller and richer. Further, when women acutely feel the emptiness of the nest as the children leave, there is often great compensation, as well as comfort, in being wanted and needed by their partner.

In fact, Gail Sheehay, in *Passages,* noted a steep rise of contentment in the sexual act when couples reach their forties, leveling off at a higher plateau after fifty. And the editors of the Consumers Union Report, *Love, Sex and Aging,* summarizing 4,246 responses to a survey of "older" Americans, noted that "the panorama of love, sex, and aging here presented is far richer and more diverse than the stereotype of life after fifty, or than the view presented by earlier studies of aging. Both the quality and the quantity of sexual activity reported can properly be described as astonishing."[2]

Strength and energy are reduced as we grow older, Masters and Johnson noted in *Human Sexual Response,* but this does not significantly limit orgasm. In fact, women in good health can continue having orgasms until very late in life, even well into the eighties. Since the male erection can often be maintained longer (both because of experience and changing physiology), his performance and effectiveness from the woman's point of view may actually improve.

Some women worry specifically that their sex drive will diminish as their estrogen level drops and, indeed, this concern may also be felt by their husbands. One gentleman mourned to us that his fifty-eight-year-old wife "is no longer a woman."

Well, he's wrong. There is no clear indication that a woman's libido is dependent upon her estrogen level. (However, loss of the male hormone, testosterone, in a man does lead to impotence.)

Actually, a woman's androgens, produced by both the

ovaries and the adrenals, seem to play a more important role than estrogen in sexual responsiveness. Younger women who have an oophorectomy (surgical removal of uterus and ovaries) and also removal of the adrenal glands, thus eliminating androgens, will experience a sharp decline in libido. Likewise, the pituitary gland, if obliterated, will inhibit the production of androgens, and libido markedly declines. But estrogen has not been felt to be essential to libido.

Many women also seem to feel anxious about what amount of sexual activity is normal at this time of life. We feel that what's comfortable for both you and your partner is right. What Masters and Johnson or any other researchers quote as the norm should not be important to you. Whether intercourse occurs once or twice a week, or once a month, the sole criteria should be that you're both comfortable with your sexual expression.

No matter what the frequency, we would urge you to remember the tremendous human need for closeness. In the much-publicized survey by columnist Ann Landers, she asked her women readers, "Would you be content to be held close and treated tenderly, and forget about 'the act'?" Of the more than 90,000 women who replied, a whopping 64,000 chorused, "Yes!" Surprisingly, 40 percent of the yea-voters were under age forty. In sometimes impassioned prose, they expressed dissatisfaction with their mates' lovemaking and a desire for more human contact. It should be noted, however, that the 28 percent who answered, "No!" were as fervent in their replies as the yes-sayers.

Researchers caution that a survey of this sort tends to be self-selective, that people who have a problem are more likely to respond. Still, the sad implication to us is that so many women evidently have been unable to communicate their unhappiness to their spouses. As Ann Landers wrote in a subsequent column, "Women must tell their men what they want—and men need to listen and do their best to deliver."[3]

It is so important to nurture tenderness and touching for there are always times when intercourse isn't possible or mutually desirable. That doesn't mean that you and your husband are not in love or not happy, or that you have no sexuality or a poor marriage. Do not underestimate the closeness of hugs, kisses, cuddling, holding. They're some of the most important aspects of your physical expression of love.

One woman expressed it this way, "My husband and I have a more special, intimate relationship than ever before. It doesn't seem to have so much to do with sex per se. It's just that wonderful closeness."

Orene found a similar outlook as she advised a patient named Ruth, the wife of a university professor. Ruth suffered from a combination of problems, including lack of estrogen and a skin condition of the vulva. Her pain during and after intercourse was so intense that she and her husband had stopped having intercourse. They still had a close and secure relationship, however, and as Orene talked with Ruth, it became evident that Orene was more concerned about Ruth's ability to have intercourse than she was.

Her symptoms are now gone, and she is working on reconditioning to relax and know that pain will not be the main sensation. The couple's continued closeness has prevailed as more important to both of them than the act of intercourse itself. If one person is dissatisfied, however, the matter needs to be dealt with through compromise and, often, through counseling or relationship-building.

Problems may arise, too, when one spouse has a heart attack or an episode of illness limiting physical expression of sexuality for a time. Couples often react with fear and are reluctant to initiate intercourse again—particularly patients with heart problems. There certainly is a time when intercourse could be unhealthy, but the risks are usually very small after the recuperation period and, with little modification, most doctors favor a return to normal sexual practices.

In fact, they point to a number of benefits from intercourse, including pleasure, exhilaration, release of tension, mild exercise, and a sense of well-being. There does seem to be some truth to the old "use it or lose it" adage. Many sexologists state that consistency of sexual relations is the key to continuously vigorous sexual expression both for the man and the woman.

There is some medical support for this view. For example, when there is routine dilatation of the vagina, it seems to prevent the shortening and narrowing, which can occur in postmenopausal women who are not having regular intercourse. However, no matter how frequent the sexual activity, thinning of the vaginal tissues, which is the result of the loss of estrogen, will occur in some but not all women. This condition can be reversed with estrogen therapy, as we mentioned in the last chapter.

Still, an incredible number of women say to Orene, "I can't remember the last time we had intercourse."

WHY DOES SEXUAL LIFE SOMETIMES DIMINISH?

Mind over Body

You've heard, perhaps, that the biggest problem area in sexual relationships lies above the neck. Though the mind can affect us at any age, we think it's especially true during and after menopause. Whatever we believe to be true about our sexuality—the best, the worst, or somewhere in between—can become a self-fulfilling prophecy.

Sometimes, those of us who are Christians become locked into rather puritanical ideas. One is a sense of shame about the body. These negative feelings may be compounded by the fact that we have lost our girlish figures. Confessed one woman, "Every time I finish showering and pull back the curtain I see myself in the bathroom mirror. Let's face it. It's not a pretty sight!"

But let us ask: Is the body good? We believe that it is, because God has told us it is good. Not just part of it; all of it. As the creation of God, it is something special: a marvelous, working design which, despite any lumps, spots, or wrinkles, is beautiful. We are created in His image, no matter what our stage of life.

Too often the middle-aged woman tries too hard to "stay young." Some wear all-too-mod styles with extremely short skirts or a tight fit that reveals the changes in their bodies. Yet if we recognize the changes brought about by growing older and consider them when we choose our clothes, we look at ease with who we are.

Another puritanical idea, which may persist, is the concept that all sex is related to procreation. ("Be fruitful and multiply," the Lord directed.) This view of life leaves a tremendous gap in accepting one's healthy sexual expression before and after the reproductive years. A damaging outlook that may partially be an offshoot of this is to view sexual relations after fifty as lustful, as in the expression, "a dirty old man."

These concepts clearly are not biblical, as we see in the lives of Abraham and Sarah who continued an active sexual life long past the normal reproductive years. For though she had "ceased to be . . . after the manner of women," Sarah did conceive and bear a child when she was ninety and her husband a hundred!

David W. Augsburger was quoted in *For Women Only* as saying that the sex act is "perhaps the highest and most concentrated expression of love humanly possible."[4] Christ states in Matthew 19:5 that "The two shall become one flesh." As we mature, this union becomes more than ever a vital reunion, as we once again give ourselves and lose ourselves to one another. It is a coming together in the most intimate, self-forgetful sharing, which transcends all mere words or other expressions of oneness.

How grateful we should be to God for providing us with

this communion which allows us to "know" one another in the deepest, truest, most loving way imaginable!

When men or women view the middle years as "reaching the last stages of life," they may feel such psychic trauma that their sexual responses and abilities become inhibited. We hope that attitude belongs to generations past and that you and your husband are too busy setting new goals to let yourselves languish sexually at such a tender age.

Sometimes, however, there are specific physical problems which inhibit sexual activity. Unfortunately, many women don't feel free to express them. We talked recently with a man who lamented the end of a "marvelous sex life, after my wife had her uterus and ovaries removed." The man's wife had admitted to her sister that intercourse had become painful to her, but evidently she wasn't comfortable telling either her husband or her physician. What a pity, because she (and he) most certainly could be helped.

Painful Intercourse

Nothing is less conducive to lovemaking than pain. Some women find it to be most acute at the beginning of intercourse. Some experience a great deal of discomfort afterwards and may have persistent symptoms for a day or so. Usually the pain is described as a feeling of "rawness, like an abrasion," which may continue as a burning pain that is not easily relieved and can grow until it's literally impossible to have intercourse.

Once pain is experienced, it starts a cycle: the pain leads to feelings of dissatisfaction, the dissatisfaction leads to tension over further intercourse, the tension leads to more pain. After a period of conditioning, you'll associate intercourse so closely with pain that you'll want to avoid it. You feel confused and inadequate and guilty so you reject these unpleasant feelings by avoiding the cause, intercourse.

There are three things to look for when pain occurs:

yeast and bacterial infections; an external problem, such as chronic vulvitis; and loss of estrogen to the tissues. There's no reason to suffer silently with any of these physical problems.

A *yeast infection* is an overgrowth of a fungus called "monilia," and is characterized by itching, burning, discharge, and sometimes, painful intercourse. The body always contains this yeast, which is the same as bread yeast, but at times the body's resistance diminishes and the fungus multiplies. Typically this happens when the tissues are already irritated (as in the thinning from a lack of estrogen). But it also occurs in a hot climate and with failure to allow the vulva or external genital areas to "breathe." Be wary of wearing pantyhose or slacks continuously.

The treatment for yeast infection is the application of antifungal vaginal creams. Prevention may be possible by eating or drinking foods which contain acidophilus bacteria, such as yogurt, buttermilk, and acidophilus milk. Although these bacteria are normally found in large numbers in the vagina, if they're depleted, as they can be when you take antibiotics, the stage is set to allow yeast to multiply. Douching with yogurt can increase these "good" bacteria in the vagina.

Bacterial vaginitis occurs when *hemophilus vaginalis* (a bacteria commonly found in the vagina of healthy patients) multiplies out of control. It can be associated with discomfort and discharge, but by far the most disturbing symptom is an overpowering fishy odor. This smell can be extremely disturbing to your feeling of cleanliness, and the odor becomes exaggerated during intercourse.

A patient of Orene's who was separated from her husband felt that this was a primary cause for his leaving. She felt the odor was sometimes noticeable even at work. The condition is treatable with antibiotics, but it can recur.

Vulvitis, the inflammation of the external sexual organs, is not caused by lack of estrogens and will not respond to estrogen replacement. It can be an allergy to soaps or to nylon underwear and will respond to steroid creams such as Vali-sone.

If there is any question about the irritation, however, a biopsy of the tissue is important, because at times a precancer can mimic a chronic vulvitis. Both can contribute to discomfort during intercourse.

The first two conditions discussed above are not limited to the menopausal years, but the third cause of painful intercourse is.

Atrophic vaginitis is related to loss of estrogen, which both dries and thins the tissues. About 30 per cent of menopausal women report painful intercourse relating to poor lubrication, pain with penetration, or pain after intercourse. These problems may relate to decreasing function of the lubricating glands (the Bartholin's glands, located at the opening of the vagina); narrowing of the introitus or opening of the vagina; or thinning, narrowing, or perhaps shortening of the vagina as an effect of estrogen loss.

This change sneaks up on women, perhaps two years or so after their last period. Not only is the vagina generally less moist, but also there's a failure to lubricate during foreplay. For some women and their husbands this looms as a distinct loss. They view the onset of vaginal lubrication as a facet of womanhood, corresponding to the erection for a man, and spontaneity may be impaired.

Interestingly, in a study of fifty-nine menopausal women at Rutgers Medical School, these symptoms did not decrease the frequency of intercourse as compared to the control women, who did not experience painful intercourse. In Orene's experience, however, this pain can become severe enough to inhibit intercourse altogether after a period of time. An extreme attitude was summed up by one woman who reported, "I said to my husband, 'Well, I feel all dried up and so do you, so let's just forget it.' "

Of course, her husband was by no means "dried up"

and surely resented this affront to his sexuality. There is specific help for her in overcoming this attitude.

Estrogen creams reverse the vaginal skin changes and make intercourse comfortable once again. Those patients who still experience pain may have learned to tighten their muscles as a response to pain. They need to recondition and teach themselves they can relax and not experience discomfort, once the tissues return to normal. This relearning process has been outlined in detail by Masters and Johnson in their book on sexual adequacy.

In the few patients who do not notice quick results with the creams, oral estrogens may be the answer. Consumers Union reports statistically that postmenopausal women taking estrogen have a higher enjoyment of sex than their sisters and may have sexual intercourse more frequently. However, it does not say there's a direct relationship to estrogen use. Although the literature has historically denied that estrogens have a major effect on libido, some of the more recent statistical studies tend to show a positive change in sexual behavior. Still, the only definite indication for replacement estrogen therapy is for treatment of vaginal dryness and atrophy in the postmenopausal years.

Lubricants such as K-Y jelly are not ideal, but they are a solution to the woman who can't use estrogen. Some women prefer such preparations as Lubifax or Transilube.

Hot Flashes

It's difficult to feel cuddly and lovable if you come up dripping wet in the midst of a warm embrace. You may simply need to be honest and call for time out. May your husband be as understanding as one patient man who, whenever he realized his wife's distress, paused and flapped the bedsheet to cool her. He also sympathetically dubbed her, "The Flasher."

Fatigue

Many menopausal women complain of fatigue and/or sleep disturbances. No wonder they're not always ready for a night of love which begins at midnight! But there *are* ways to overcome. Obviously, you can plan an "early retirement." Or what about mornings, when you're both more rested? Many couples now freed of children dashing in and out of the house, enjoy Saturday "matinees." This stage in life is a time when you may well want to modify prior patterns.

Low Level of Fitness

There's no question that the pleasure of sexual relations is enhanced by a fit body, which results from the three-pronged approach of sufficient exercise, a balanced diet, and adequate sleep.

Both you and your husband should follow a program of regular exercise. Perhaps you can do it together (see chapter 6 for specific suggestions). And by the way, intercourse itself is an "exercise" which many couples believe keeps them feeling active and vigorous. The oxygen usage in the sex act is about the same as in climbing one or two flights of stairs.

In your diet, strive toward eliminating the "empty calories" of rich, sugar-laden foods and concentrate on a balance of protein, milk products, cereals and grains, vegetables and fruits. The Superintendent of Documents, Government Printing Office, Washington, D.C. 20402, offers several low-cost booklets on eating well.

And finally, if it's difficult for you to get sufficient sleep at night, schedule naps for yourself during the day if you can, or on weekends even if they cut into your list of to-be-done's. Most husbands would readily trade a rested "you" for an immaculate house, a perfect dinner party, or a weed-free garden.

Male Midlife Crisis

If a man experiences an after-forty, so-called "male menopause," it will sometimes manifest itself in his sexual life, perhaps in increased sexual drive, but sometimes in malfunction. He may suddenly be faced with premature ejaculation, or may find himself unable to achieve or sustain an erection. Since it's been pointed out that after forty a man's most important sex organ is his brain, you can play a vital role in reassuring him of his manhood, your love for him, and that, like menopause, "this, too, will pass."

Moreover, many, if not most men, long for a wife who is more sexually aggressive. Although this is probably *not* the time for you to become overwhelmingly dominant, perhaps you can take a subtly more active role in foreplay and intercourse.

WHAT IF YOU JUST DON'T FEEL LIKE IT?

Generally, men are more likely than women to wish for more sex. So there may be times when your husband's desire is obvious, but you can think of a dozen things you'd rather do, including sleep or maybe even (but we hope not) housework! Sometimes you may need to negotiate another specific time.

Others will find enormous rewards in sacrificing just a little for their husbands. During a time in life when it's easy to become absorbed in what *you* are feeling, it's good to stop and take your eyes off yourself. Almost certainly, in pleasing your husband, you yourself will find pleasure. Remember, too, some men are not very adept at expressing closeness apart from sex. It's a closeness you particularly need at this time, which helps to give you a special sense of self-worth. So don't, whatever you do, give it up.

If you're tempted to plead the proverbial headache, you

might learn from one woman who very sensibly takes her feelings to God. "Lord," she prays, "You know this isn't my idea, and I don't feel very loving. So I am going to claim *Your* love and ask You to allow it to flow through me." This attitude of trust is helpful in sexual love.

Another way of increasing your mutual satisfaction which, in turn, may increase your desire, is to practice the Kegel exercises described in chapter 4 for treatment of urinary incontinence. The method is simply to contract the internal muscles as in stopping urination. These exercises strengthen not just the muscles surrounding the urinary tract, but also the vaginal muscles.

Contracting these muscles a few times just before intercourse seems to set the stage for the involuntary contraction of these muscles in sexual climax. And contracting the muscles during intercourse not only facilitates your reaching orgasm, but it also enhances your husband's pleasure. Particularly if there are problems with impotence, contraction of the vaginal muscles helps you accommodate the partially erect penis.

WHAT CAN YOUR HUSBAND DO TO HELP YOU?

No matter how sympathetic your husband may be, he will never completely understand what you are going through. But he won't understand at all if you don't *tell* him how you feel and what you need. We don't mean issuing long and repeated lists of woes and complaints. But we do mean explaining if, for instance, you're feeling a bit fragile and vulnerable during these changes, and if you have some particular desires. In a sense, you're like the little girl whose mother warned her before they entered the candy shop not to ask the owner for a gumdrop. Just as they were about to leave, another mother came in with her daughter, who promptly pointed at the jar of gumdrops and asked, "Can I have one?" The owner immediately gave a piece of candy to her.

"You see?" the first little girl said to her mother. "If you don't ask for it, you don't get it!"

Remember, too, your husband may be fearful of causing you pain, which is all the more reason to help him understand what will be helpful to you. If you would appreciate a little more conversational sharing of your lives beforehand, or if you now feel you need longer foreplay, by all means tell him in a loving way.

If you have difficulty talking about it, perhaps this would be a good time to suggest that together you review the anatomy and physiology of sexual response. Masters and Johnson's *Human Sexual Response,* the Consumers Union Report titled *Love, Sex and Aging,* or the LaHayes' *The Act of Marriage* may be helpful. If you and your spouse cannot talk and the problems seem insurmountable, remember, there are numerous people who can counsel you, including your minister, psychologists, and in some urban areas, sexual therapists.

And you might wish to ask your husband to pray with you. In *The Act of Marriage,* Tim and Beverly LaHaye report that "many spiritual Christians pray before going to bed."[5] And indeed, the act of committing this time to your Creator seems an altogether appropriate focus. It also takes both your husband's eyes and yours off your "performance," freeing both of you to enjoy this God-ordained union.

"He Isn't Interested"

Orene occasionally has a patient who comes to her and says, "My husband is just not interested in sex. In fact, we haven't had relations in months. I don't think anything's wrong with him, and I don't understand what's happening."

There are usually two different reasons for such a change. One may be that he has some emotional depression, but a wife will usually know if things aren't going well for him. Or, difficult as it is to face, there is also a strong possibility that he is finding his sexual outlet in another place, either in a homosexual relationship or with another woman.

Many women go to the point of divorce, not realizing what is happening and, truly, even their best friend won't tell them. It's such a difficult thing to reveal! This possibility is Orene's first concern when a patient tells of her husband's disinterest in sex. So she will ask, "Is it possible your husband has a relationship outside your marriage?"

The usual response is, "Oh, no! I don't think so."

The wife may simply be naive, or she may not want to know. Denial is sometimes the mind's way of coping with the problem.

Before leaping to conclusions, however, it's important to consider if there could be any physical condition which might reduce the male libido. Tranquilizers and some blood pressure medications can specifically decrease the sexual desire and, in some cases, produce impairment. If this is the case, it might be worthwhile to consult with a physician about an alternative drug that would not produce the same side-effects.

THE SINGLES SCENE

In the world today, the assumption prevails that *everybody,* married or single, has a sexual life, and that, if you're divorced or widowed, you couldn't possibly live without it.

It's important to accept your sexuality, but it doesn't mean you must embrace the world's values. You may not desire to form another sexual relationship, but to find fulfillment in other ways, through your work, your children, your church, your relationship with the Lord. Will you believe that your God is sufficient to meet all your needs, as He stated in Philippians 4:19?

Masturbation as an outlet, though not biblically forbidden, is not encouraged by many churches, which believe God instilled the sex drive in humans, not for self-gratification, but to inspire them to mate through marriage. From a medical standpoint, however, we can say that masturbation has never been found to be harmful. (No, it doesn't cause blindness!)

On the other hand, you may feel a tremendous need for closeness, and eventually will remarry. Generally you can look forward to a smooth transition to a new sexual relationship.

We hope this chapter has dispelled some of your blues if you feel like the menopausal wife who complained, "It just seems like sex is one more thing in my life that isn't working."

It can and will get better, so don't give up! Don't be afraid to express your problems to your doctor and to ask for his or her help. Then you, like so many people in your age group, will understand what the book, *Sex after Sixty*, refers to as "the second language of sex." Among the various meanings of love and sex it lists are the opportunity for expression of passion; affection; admiration; loyalty and other positive emotions; an affirmation of one's body and its functioning; the pleasure of being touched or caressed; a sense of romance and an affirmation of life.[6] We pray that you and your partner may "speak" this language well for many years to come.

Chapter Seven

HOW TO AVOID
DOWAGER'S HUMP

"My mother once was a stunning woman," a forty-year-old daughter remembered. "Now she's a bent-over little old lady who can't even hold her head erect. I look at her and sometimes I wonder: am I looking at myself, twenty-five years from now?"

The answer to this woman's question does not have to be yes. Today we know that osteoporosis (brittle bone disease, which caused the mother's stooped posture) can be prevented. A little foresight can make a difference.

Women today can expect to live 78.3 years. If you are over thirty-five, you are truly in the middle of your life, not on the way downhill as some suggest. The next four decades of your life will be affected by how you care for your body now.

We hear some people say not to worry. "Whatever will be, will be." Is this good stewardship of the bodies God gave us? If we see our bodies as temples in which God lives, as Paul describes them in I Corinthians 6:19, we'll want to be the best possible caretakers.

Why not follow Solomon's suggestion: Be a prudent person who "foresees the difficulties ahead and prepares for them," rather than a "simpleton (who) goes blindly on and suffers the consequences" (Proverbs 22:3 TLB).

OSTEOPOROSIS, A MAJOR PROBLEM

Let's look at the magnitude of osteoporosis and see what we can do to forestall it.

Many of us thought that the bent-over-little-old-lady syndrome was an inevitable part of aging until articles began to appear in newspapers and magazines a few years ago about osteoporosis. With the "graying" of our population, with more than 32 million women over age fifty in the United States, this disease (which results in life-threatening bone fractures) is reaching epidemic proportions and is a major health issue.

It is so serious that Dr. Robert Butler, Pulitzer Prize winning author and former head of the National Institute on Aging, termed it one of the "polios" of geriatrics.

The difficulty with osteoporosis is that it is so insidious. Most women don't know they have it until they break a bone, and then it's too late to reverse the disease. Yet osteoporosis afflicts twenty-five percent of white women over age sixty; by age seventy-five, fifty percent of women are affected. And of those women who experience a surgical menopause *without* hormone replacement, fifty-nine percent will suffer from osteoporosis.

We saw in chapter 3 that osteoporosis manifests itself most commonly in fractures of the hip, the vertebrae, and the wrist (which is called a Colles' fracture). Hip fractures are the most disabling and life threatening. Half of all women over sixty-five have detectable wedging (a break of the vertebrae, in which the front but not the back section of the vertebrae collapses), and ten percent have at least one totally collapsed vertebra. These fractures can cause pain, height loss of as much as eight inches, pronounced stooping, and a dowagers' hump. Fractures of the wrist, usually as the result of a fall, are ten times more common in postmenopausal women than in men over the age of fifty, but they usually heal without any lasting problems.

Our bones are living tissue and constantly undergo a process of remodeling, that is, building new bone tissue and resorption or tearing-down of old tissue. A positive balance of building bone tissue to replace old tissue prevails until age thirty to thirty-five. Then, since estrogen has a role in bone-rebuilding, when a woman stops producing estrogen the bone loss accelerates. In fact, for the first five to six years after menopause a woman loses bone six times as rapidly as does a man; but around age sixty-five, her rate of bone loss begins to slow and become similar to a man's. When this loss reaches a point where the bones become porous or honeycombed and weak, and they begin to fracture.

There are two kinds of bone tissue, cortical (the hard, outer layer) and trabecular (the spongy bone that lines the marrow). Different bones have different percentages of cortical and trabecular bone. The first to be affected in osteoporosis is the porous trabecular bone. Women in their sixties may suffer from wedging, a fracture of the vertebrae, which contain more trabecular bone. Hip fractures occur later in life, because this bony tissue contains a large amount of cortical bone, which is unaffected by the disease until later.

DIAGNOSING POTENTIAL PROBLEMS

If you have thin, fragile bones to begin with, you obviously will be in more danger. Black women naturally have denser bone structure, so although they also experience bone loss after menopause, they are not as likely to suffer osteoporosis as are Oriental and white women, especially those who are petite and have delicate frames. If you also have blue eyes and transparent skin through which your veins tend to show, or if you smoke, you are at still greater risk. If you have had your ovaries removed or experienced an early menopause, or if your mother, grandmother, or sister had osteoporosis you are even more likely to have osteoporosis.

Your diet can increase the possibility of your getting this disease, since caffeine, alcohol, protein, and phosphate in excess accelerate bone loss. Too little calcium is a common

OSTEOPOROSIS

Common Bones Affected	-% Trabecular/ Cortical Bone	Type of Fracture
1. Vertebrae (Thoracic T-8-L-3—upper back	90% 10%	Wedging, then collapse of vertebrae
		Usually occurs 15-20 years after menopause
2. Hip	50% 50%	Fracture of upper femur or leg bone Usually occurs 20-40 years after menopause
3. Forearm	25% 75%	Colles' fracture
		Usually occurs 10-15 years after menopause

cause of osteoporosis. Certain medical illnesses increase the risk: diabetes, rheumatoid arthritis, hyperthyroidism, kidney disease, and Cushing's Syndrome (an overgrowth of basophilic cells of the pituitary, which is characterized by obesity and muscular weakness).

An easy way to detect bone loss is to measure your height regularly. One inch of height is lost with each compression fracture of the vertebrae. Most people do lose a little height in aging, perhaps a quarter or half an inch, but losses of an inch or more are generally the result of vertebral fracture. If you're getting shorter, you may already be suffering from osteoporosis.

Another way to detect impending bone loss is to ask your dentist to check for bone loss in your jaw. Many dentists use a callibrated probe to measure from the top of the gum to where it attaches to the bone. As the gum diminishes, so, often, does the bone. Your dentist can tell you if he perceives bone loss in the jaw. If he does, pay attention, for loss here, in what has been described as the body's "most active bone," usually precedes bone loss in other parts of the body.

Single photon absorptiometry is the best inexpensive way to measure bone loss in your body. A densitometer measures the mineral content in the bones of the forearm by calculating how many gamma rays are absorbed. The more absorption, the greater the bone mineral content. This method can detect a one-to-three percent loss of bone, while an x-ray does not show a problem until there is a thirty percent loss. This painless test takes less than ten minutes and exposes you to less than one-hundredth the amount of radiation of an ordinary arm x-ray.

At the Center for Climacteric Studies in Gainesville, single photon absorptiometry has been used successfully for screening patients without symptoms, including those who have less than an average amount of bone mass at skeletal maturity (age thirty-five). It is also effective for monitoring women on treatment every three, six, or twelve months to determine their progress. In addition, a mobile densitometer travels from the Center throughout the state in a growing screening program for osteoporosis.

Unfortunately this equipment is not available everywhere, but at a cost of about twenty thousand dollars, it would be a valuable addition to any medical center. We look forward to the day when women throughout the country will have access to this testing.

Once a baseline measurement is made, subsequent testing on a regular basis determines whether or not bone mineral content remains constant or is diminishing. Although osteoporosis cannot be reversed, early bone loss can be prevented. That is why it's so important to detect bone loss before it reaches the point of osteoporosis. In fact, the Center for Climacteric Studies stresses the importance of regular tests for bone mass, beginning in your thirties and forties.

(Dr. Morris Notelovitz, director of the Center for Climacteric Studies at Gainesville, Florida, is a pioneer in detecting and preventing osteoporosis. His book, *Stand Tall,* details his work and findings and is an invaluable aid if you'd like to know more about the disease.)

The only drawback to the single photon absorptiometry method is that it does not always correlate accurately with changes in bone mass in the spine. The Computerized Axial Tomography (CAT) scan, a method for viewing cross sections of bone with x-rays, gives the most accurate determination of this bone loss. Certain hospitals are beginning to use CAT scans as a screening device. Baseline measurements are taken, and women come back every six to twelve months to see if they're gaining or losing bone mass or holding their own.

The disadvantage of CAT scanning is that it does expose you and your internal organs to relatively high levels of radiation, and it is more expensive (one hundred-ninety dollars for each scan in one southern California hospital).

Dual photon absorptiometry also shows promise for identifying women at risk for spinal problems, but it is available only in research and in a few clinical centers.

If there is testing available in your area, and especially if you are in the high risk group, take advantage of the screening in order to keep your later years healthy. If it's not available, we strongly suggest that you assume you may develop osteoporosis and follow the preventative measures we'll outline in the following section.

PREVENTION OF OSTEOPOROSIS

Yes, you really can protect yourself against osteoporosis! There are three ways to do it: get enough calcium, exercise, and add hormone therapy.

You've heard that we never outgrow our need for milk. More accurately, we never outgrow our need for the calcium it provides. Unfortunately, milk products are often the first to be eliminated when a woman counts calories. Thus the average American woman consumes only 45 milligrams of calcium each day. But the recommended daily allowance (RDA) for adults is 800 milligrams. Menopausal and post-menopausal women need more, 1400 to 1500 milligrams.

There are 290 milligrams of calcium in eight ounces of milk, and you can use nonfat milk if you're watching your weight and/or cholesterol. Hard cheeses, such as cheddar, Swiss, and brick, are fine calcium sources and are better than soft cheeses like cottage cheese. Also good are green vegetables (broccoli, collards, kale, mustard, and turnip greens), nuts, red salmon, sardines, and dried beans. Another excellent source is tofu, that amazing high protein, low fat, no-cholesterol, cheeselike food, which is made from soybeans. One restaurant owner calls tofu "the food of the future." Yoghurt is a fine calcium source, too, and may be tolerated by women who can't drink milk due to lactose intolerance.

Of course, calcium supplements are available, but absorption is limited, even when you take large amounts. Our first recommendation, then, is that you make a concerted effort to boost the calcium in your diet. If you'll look at the following table of foods and their calcium content, you'll see it isn't as difficult as you might think to get 1400 milligrams of calcium from your diet alone. For instance, three eight-ounce glasses of milk, an ounce of Swiss cheese, a cup of broccoli, and a half cup of pudding or yoghurt would do it. You'll find a number of other possible combinations as you study the table.

If you simply can't get adequate calcium from your diet, try the supplements, but be sure to read the label to see exactly how much *calcium* the different supplements contain. You'll find that there's a great difference between 1000 milligrams of calcium carbonate, which contains 400 milligrams of calcium, and calcium lactate, which contains 130 milligrams of calcium. Calcium carbonate is less expensive and gives you the most calcium per tablet. Some people chew four Tums tablets as a supplement. (Tums *are* calcium carbonate, but most other antacids are not.) This dosage does not generally create problems with the digestive system, although some women may develop constipation. Bone meal and dolomite are high in calcium, but they may be contaminated with toxic metals. Try to take your supplement between meals, and save a third until bedtime, since it's best absorbed when your body's at rest.

Incidentally, some women are afraid that calcium causes kidney stones. If you stay under 2000 milligrams a day, you're at very minimal risk. However, if you've had a problem with kidney stones, check with your doctor before taking calcium supplements.

Remember, vitamin D is important for the forming of new bones and metabolizing calcium, so be sure you are getting the recommended daily allowance of 400 international units. Some of the calcium supplements already have vitamin D. Sunshine also provides it, but it is more difficult to measure.

How early in the climacteric should you start increasing your calcium intake? If you are in an at risk group, you should not wait until menopause but should begin at about age thirty-five with 1000 milligrams a day.

Although your daily intake of calcium is adequate, you need to consider other factors because a number of other foods and medications can affect your calcium balance. Dr. Notelovitz calls these "bone robbers," foods that actually increase calcium excretion or decrease absorption. One bone robber is protein, a part of your diet that is necessary. If you want to maintain your calcium balance, it's important to avoid an excess of protein. Forty-four grams, which is about the recommended daily intake of protein, equals about two

CALCIUM CONTENT OF SELECTED FOODS

Food	Amount	Calcium (mg.)
Dairy Products		
Skim Milk	1 c.	288
Whole Milk	1 c.	296
Swiss cheese	1 cu. in.*	139
Cheddar cheese	1 cu. in	129
Parmesan cheese (grated)	1 Tbsp.	68
Cottage cheese	6 oz.	160
Yoghurt		
(whole milk)	1 c.	272
(skim milk)	1 c.	294
Ice cream	1 c.	194
Ice milk	1 c.	204
Ice milk (soft serve)	1 c.	273
Pudding		
chocolate	1 c.	250
vanilla	1 c.	298
Meat, poultry, seafood		
Beef	2 ½ oz.	10
Chicken breast	2 ½	9
Eggs, whole	1	27
Oysters, raw	1 c.	226
Salmon	3 oz.	167
Sardines	3 oz.	372
Tuna	3 oz.	7
Nuts		
Almonds	½ c.	160
Pecans	½ c.	42
Walnuts	½ c.	50
Fruits, Vegetables		
Orange	1 med.	54
Rhubarb	1 c. ckd.	212
Strawberries	1 c.	31
Asparagus	1 c.	37

Beans		
Lima	1 c.	80
Green	1 c.	72
Broccoli	1 stalk	158
Carrots	1 c.	45
Greens, ckd.		
Collard	1 c.	289
Turnip	1 c.	252
Mustard	1 c.	193
Peanuts		
(roasted)	1 c.	107
Peas, green	1 c.	44
Spinach	1 c.	200
Squash	1 c.	55
Tomatoes	1 med.	24
Tofu	3½ oz.	128
Grain products		
Bran flakes		
w. raisins	1 c.	28
Bread	1 slice	23
Cake		
(from mix)	1 piece	55
Pancakes		
(plain,		
buttermilk)	1 cake	58
Pizza w.	5½ in.	
cheese	section	107
Waffle	1	179
(from mix)		

*cubic inches

(List derived from Krause, M.V., and Hahan, L. K. Food, *Nutrition and Diet Therapy.* Philadelphia: W. B. Saunders Co., 1979, p. 828.)

hamburgers and is enough to cause bone loss, one study has shown.

Salt also increases excretion of calcium in the urine. Two grams, which is only one teaspoon per day, can accelerate calcium excretion. Coffee robs you of calcium, as does fiber, especially fiber derived from cereal. Of course, fiber is essential to your diet, so don't try to eliminate it. But try not to mix it with high calcium foods, because it does decrease the absorption of calcium in the intestine.

It's also important to watch the ratio of calcium to phosphorus in your diet. High phosphorus foods are red meat, cola drinks, brewer's yeast, and, of course, processed foods with phosphorus additives. You should probably limit foods that are high in phosphorus and low in calcium. It's also better to eat more vegetables and white meats, such as fish or poultry.

"Bone robbers" obviously should not be eliminated from your diet, but be careful of consuming them in excess. Also, a basic understanding of how these foods interplay can help you in your diet and menu planning.

We are in the process of learning more about the effects of foods on our health, with research studies showing such positive factors as a decrease in hypertension with high calcium diets, a decrease in colon cancer with less red meats and higher fiber intake. But we have yet to put our facts into a total perspective, so we can present an ideal diet for each individual. We hope more "customized" diets will be possible in future years. Meanwhile, the old theme of moderation seems pertinent when you consider foods that decrease calcium absorption or utilization.

In addition, be wary of certain medications that stimulate bone loss. These include steroids and the many antacids that contain aluminum. (Those that are acceptable are Alka Seltzer, Alka-2, Bisodol, Cirocarbonate, Eno, Marblen, Percy Medicine, Titralac, and Tums.)

It has also been shown that smoking and drinking alcohol in excess are associated with accelerated bone loss, which is only one of many reasons they should be eliminated.

Exercise!

If your calcium intake is in balance, can you rest on your laurels? Definitely not. In fact, we hope you don't rest at all. We know that bone atrophy, or wasting away of the bone, results from inactivity, regardless of how much calcium is given. We saw this result in the study of astronauts on Gemini flights IV, V, and VII. Bone atrophy occurred even though the astronauts had adequate dietary calcium. In another study, three young men on a controlled diet and at bedrest for thirty-six weeks showed a thirty-nine percent decrease in bone mineral content of their heel bones. Resumption of normal activity reversed the bone loss, but a similar amount of time was required for replacement.

Just as chronic inactivity results in bone loss, chronic activity produces bone gain. Numerous studies of athletes indicate that bone mass increases in the specific area of greatest stress. The thickness of bone in a male professional tennis players' dominant arm was 34.9 percent greater than in the nondominant arm. Intercollegiate women swimmers and tennis players had greater bone mineral content at two sites in the arm than nonswimmers and nontennis players. But there was no significant difference between the lumbar spine densities of swimmers and the control groups, while tennis players showed a 20.25 percent greater lumbar density than controls.

What is the difference? *Weightbearing exercise* builds bone mass. This conclusion is based on a number of studies, including research over the past five years at the University of Wisconsin by Everett L. Smith, Ph.D., who directs the Biogerontology Laboratory of the Department of Preventive Medicine. His work includes following 200 women between ages thirty-five and sixty-five (80 in a control group, 120 in a physical activity group) for a three-to four-year period.

Smith concluded that bone responds dynamically to stress by increases in mass and changes in geometric characteristics. He believes, too, that exercise may also have a strengthening effect on the bone beyond the increase in bone mass. He found that the bone mineral mass of exercising animals was not different from that of controls in a current study, but the strength of their bones was significantly enhanced.

Research also suggests that exercise benefits animals by increasing the blood flow to the bones, producing small electrical potentials in the bone tissue, which stimulate bone growth.

Noting that the major areas endangered by osteoporosis are the femur (hip), spine, and wrist, Smith recommends that exercise programs include activities of muscular and weightbearing activities for all three areas, as well as aerobic activities, such as walking or jogging. And by the way, Smith's research indicates it's never too late for your bones to benefit from exercise. A study of aging females (sixty-nine to ninety-five years old) demonstrated increased bone mineral as the result of increased physical activity.

Which forms of exercise are best for your bones? The answer is weight-bearing activities that stress the long bones of the body, such as walking, jogging, hiking, biking, rowing, and jumping rope. As Everett Smith suggests, you might want to add specific upper body exercise, such as swimming, to those activities that do not stress arm bones.

We'll soon learn more about the bone-building benefits of various types of exercise from an on-going program at the Center for Climacteric Studies. This study monitors bone mass of women who walk on treadmills, both with and without backpacks, and groups riding bicycles and using Nautilus weight-training equipment.

Incidentally, have you wondered why obese women are less likely to suffer from osteoporosis? It's not just because their fat tissues convert androgens to estrogen, but also because their weight stresses the bones, causing formation of new bone to meet the stress.

Hormone replacement

The facts are clear: Postmenopausal bone loss is the direct consequence of the body's loss of estrogens. A dosage of .625 milligrams of Premarin a day or the equivalent in other forms of estrogen during menopause will prevent osteoporosis. However, women on estrogen therapy should still pay attention to calcium intake. They need the same amount as premenopausal women, 1000 milligrams per day, while women not taking estrogen need 1400.

How long should estrogen be continued? Doctors are not sure, but it may be until about age sixty-five. We do know, however, that it should be started within three years after menopause begins. Even if it's started within six years after menopause, further loss of bone mass will be prevented. The Consensus Development Conference on Osteoporosis held by the National Institute in 1984 carefully stated that "there is no convincing evidence that initiating estrogen therapy in elderly women will prevent osteoporosis."

While statistics show that women on estrogen therapy sustained sixty percent fewer wrist and hip fractures and ninety percent fewer vertebral fractures, we still cannot justify every woman's taking estrogen to prevent osteoporosis. The risks must be evaluated, and since only twenty-five percent of postmenopausal women are likely to have osteoporosis, we can say that only twenty-five percent need this drug therapy to avoid this disease.

Many physicians feel the conservative approach is best, to emphasize diet and exercise, and if this fails, to go to estrogen. There must be a monitoring, however, to determine if the conservative approach will be adequate. Measurement of height, bone densitometry measurements, or perhaps CAT scanning can provide valuable guidelines for determining the presence of osteoporosis.

If you are at risk and if you're concerned about the possibility of estrogen causing cancer, remember that 40,000 women fracture their hips each year. Of these, 30 percent will die, while only 2,300 women die of endometrial cancer each year. It's clear which alternative is safer.

Remember, too, no matter what preventive measures you take for osteoporosis, they are just that, preventive, not therapeutic. There is still no evidence that women who have already developed osteoporosis will achieve bone reformation. In fact, one of the saddest situations is that of the sixty-five-year-old woman who needs hip surgery following a fracture when the x-ray shows osteoporotic bones. Someone may say, "Let's give her estrogen." But estrogen at this point will only prevent further bone loss. It will not replace lost bone.

So once osteoporosis develops, it becomes a matter of working to keep the condition from worsening rather than of treatment. Exercise could include twice-daily walks, swimming, and specific back exercises (see *Standing Tall*). And yes, estrogen and estrogen-progesterone therapy can protect you from further loss. Anabolic steroids (androgens) can also slow bone loss. Be careful with fluoride; it may increase bone mass, but it also makes bones more brittle. Also, while some vitamin D is vital, excessive doses of D can lead toward osteoporosis.

The forty-year-old woman at the beginning of this chapter who looked at her hunchbacked mother and wondered, *Will I someday look like my mother?* can take these steps to avoid the crippling effects of osteoporosis. She does not have to be a bent-over little old lady. Neither do you.

Chapter Eight

THREE OUNCES OF PREVENTION

"What scares me when I consider my family tree," patients sometimes tell Orene, "is breast cancer. My aunt died of it. So did my mother. And now my oldest sister has just had a mastectomy. Will I be next?"

The answer to this patient's question does not have to be a resounding yes, anymore than the answer to the woman who feared osteoporosis in the last chapter had to be yes. You've heard about taking "an ounce of prevention." We suggest three ounces of prevention. Osteoporosis certainly is a preventable condition as discussed in chapter 7. Cancer and heart disease are the primary killers of middle-aged people, but cancer, when identified early, can be cured and heart disease can be prevented. In this chapter we will talk about protecting against these diseases and also how to relieve symptoms of the less threatening, but nonetheless troublesome, fibrocystic breast disease.

CONTROLLING BREAST CANCER

Let's face it, breast cancer is something none of us likes to think about. Yet, oh, how we need to! The key is early detection of the smallest lesion or lump. Each of us has both the right and the responsibility to monitor our own breasts. Our goal, always, is to be the first one to detect a problem.

One of every eleven women will develop breast cancer in her lifetime, and approximately sixty-five percent are detected after the age of fifty. Breast cancer is the leading cause of cancer deaths in women of all ages and leads all other causes of death among women, aged forty to forty-four, in the United States. While many women worry about cancer of the uterus and there are 2,300 deaths a year from endometrial cancer (the lining of the uterus), 37,000 women die of breast cancer every year.

Certainly, you should be particularly vigilant if you are at risk: if your mother or sibling had breast cancer, if you've already had cancer in one breast, or if your first child was born when you were thirty-five or older. You are also at risk if you began menstruating at an early age, had a late menopause, are obese, have high dietary fat intake, or have had certain benign breast diseases.

Let Your Fingers Do the Checking

The problem with breast self-examination always has been that women don't know what they are feeling. Frequently they report, "Everything feels lumpy."

To help "educate women's fingers," a number of breast-care centers are opening around the country. One group called "MammaCare" uses lifelike simulated breasts made of silicone and extruded polymer. Hidden in the models are fixed and mobile lumps, ranging in size from a fourth-of-an-inch to an inch in diameter. With eight different models, which vary in firmness and nodularity, a model can be "matched" to the patient.

First the woman learns how to discriminate between normal and nodular breast tissue and how to distinguish the lumps in the models. She feels with the pads of three fingers in each spot at three different depths, using a circular motion. Then she uses the same technique on herself. She's shown a pattern of searching in vertical strips, covering the entire area from collarbone to lower bra line, armpit and ribs to the middle of the breastbone, using a pattern similar to mowing a yard (illustration 1). The two factors that affect survival are size of the tumor when removed (preferably less

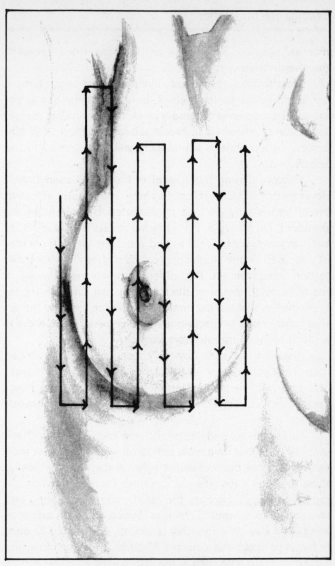

MAMMACARE METHOD OF
BREAST SELF-EXAMINATION
Illustration 1

than an inch) and whether or not the cancer has spread to the lymph nodes.

We also know that ninety-five percent of breast tumors are found by the patient herself, but the average tumor detected by a woman is just under an inch-and-a-half in diameter, *if she is untrained* in breast self-examination, and fifty percent of tumors this size already will have spread to the lymph nodes.

However, using this system of breast self-examination developed by MammaCare, women soon learn to detect breast lumps only an inch in diameter. But MammaCare president, Dr. Henry S. Pennypacker of Gainesville, Florida, believes women can learn to find much smaller lumps, ideally as small as one centimeter, or .39 inches. This early detection could mean the difference between having a mastectomy (removal of the whole breast) and a lumpectomy (removal of just the lump). It can mean catching the tumor before there is lymph-node involvement, when there is a much higher cure rate after surgery.

If you're not sure how to check your breasts, by all means ask your doctor, or see if there's a clinic in your area. You may also write to MammaCare, 900 W. 8th Ave., Gainesville, FL 32601, for information on the clinic nearest to you.

Be sure to set aside a specific time each month to check yourself. Let your menstrual period serve as a reminder for a self-check since the breasts are softer and easier to examine three to seven days after your period. Premenstrual checking is not helpful because the breast may grow lumpy and tender due to hormonal changes. When you stop menstruating, you lose your monthly reminder, and it may be easy to forget your self-examination. You may then want to establish an arbitrary date such as the first of each calendar month as the time to check yourself.

Any bloody discharge from the breast should be evaluated quickly, since it could be a sign of cancer. A clear or milky discharge, however, does not indicate a primary breast tumor, though it can suggest a hormone imbalance. Tenderness is generally thought to be associated with benign changes in the breast, especially in premenopausal women.

Of course, you will want to supplement self-examination with regular visits to your doctor. He or she may suggest additional screening, such as a mammography.

Mammography

Mammography, or x-ray pictures of the breast, identifies between eighty-five and ninety percent of small breast tumors long before they can be felt and often before they have affected the lymph nodes. The American Cancer Society now recommends a baseline mammography when you are thirty-five to fifty. After the age of fifty, mammography should be performed routinely, perhaps even yearly.

If your doctor does not plan an appropriate time to have mammography, be sure to ask about it. It is becoming a routine screening test.

Many of us are leery of this much exposure to radiation, a potential cancer cause in itself. However, the National Cancer Institute and American Cancer Society say the breasts of women aged fifty and over are much less sensitive to radiation than younger breasts, so the radiation exposure of yearly mammograms after fifty does not increase the risk of developing cancer.

Formerly we heard a good bit about thermography (measuring the body's heat variation) as a method without x-ray of measuring skin temperature to detect lumps before they can be felt. It has been shown however, to be ineffective in discovering breast cancer that is not detected by clinical exam of the breast. Therefore, it should not be substituted for mammography.

It's natural to want to avoid the possibility of unpleasant news. Such an "ostrich-with-head-in-the-sand" attitude may account for the high fatality rate of breast cancer patients. But look what you have to gain by being vigilant. Nine out of ten women treated for early breast cancer will be alive and well five years later. Be sure you persevere with monthly self-examination, in addition to visits to your doctor, and if it's recommended, periodic mammography.

FIBROCYSTIC BREAST DISEASE

A woman who finds a lump in her breast immediately thinks of cancer. But a very common benign disease called "fibrocystic breast disease" is characterized by nodularity and, often, tenderness. Sometimes there is a specific soft lump or cyst which can be aspirated (removing the fluid with a needle). If a gynecologist or surgeon aspirates a lump and can withdraw cyst fluid, the lump is benign. If not, a biopsy is indicated. Mammography is also helpful in differentiating between fibrocystic disease and a tumor. And sometimes ultrasound, or bouncing sound waves off the tissue, can be used to determine if a lump is fluid-filled.

Fortunately, you can minimize the symptoms of fibrocystic disease by eliminating certain foods and drugs that contain methylxanthines. Caffeine is a methylxanthine, which, of course, means you should eliminate coffee, tea, chocolate, and a number of soft drinks. Many over-the-counter drugs, such as Anacin and Excedrin, as well as Darvon, A.P.C. with codeine, and other prescription drugs also contain caffeine.

Some bronchial and asthma remedies, muscle relaxants, and diuretics contain the related chemicals, theophylline, and theobromine, which should also be avoided. By eliminating these substances, sixty-five percent of women with fibrocystic disease will experience relief of tenderness and lumps in one to six months. The symptoms will return, however, if caffeine is resumed.

Fortunately, fibrocystic disease is not likely to develop into breast cancer. Statistically, however, women who have biopsies for benign breast disease do have a higher rate of cancer later. But this association of increasing risk of cancer is found only in certain uncommon types of benign breast disease (which can be diagnosed only on biopsy and which your surgeon will explain).

Consider the glad tidings that fibrocystic symptoms may disappear after menopause.

PREVENTING HEART DISEASE

With Exercise

We've talked about the role of exercise in preventing osteoporosis. If you plan your exercise properly, it can also increase your cardiovascular fitness. We suggest an aerobic exercise program.

Of course, before you begin, you should check with your doctor. A stress test is also advisable. Then, be sure you start gradually. (Don't expect or try to run five miles your third week!) And *always* begin with at least five minutes of warm-up exercises and finish with five minutes of cool-down exercises.

Your goal will be to strengthen that muscle known as the heart, to get it to the point of working at seventy to eighty percent of its capacity for a period of twenty to thirty minutes, five times a week. Here is an example of how to calculate your maximal heart rate:

```
                220
minus your age:  __            Also multiply your
        = ____ total           total:  ___
        x    .70 (70%)            x    .80 (80%)
        = ___                  to   = ___


Here's an example:
                220
           - age  50
           _____
             170           170
           x 70%         x 80%
           _____      _____

        119 beats/mins. to 136 beats/min.
```

Thus at age fifty, you should aim for a 119 to 136 pulse while exercising.

Remember to check your pulse rate now and then as you exercise. Stop exercising for a moment and find your carotid artery by placing two fingers in the center of your throat under your chin. Now slide your fingers to one side into the hollow that you can feel beside your trachea or windpipe. When you locate this pulse, count it for ten seconds and multiply by six. If it's more than your maximal heart rate you're working too hard and should slow down. If it's below, push yourself a little harder.

All of the forms of exercise we've mentioned for preventing osteoporosis—walking, jogging, rowing, hiking, biking, skipping rope—are excellent cardiovascular conditioners. So, too, are swimming and some forms of "dancercize." (If you'd like more information about exercise, you might want to read a book such as *Aerobics for Women* by Mildred and Ken Cooper.)

Interestingly, of all the exercise programs in the study at the Center for Climacteric Studies, brisk walking (here on a treadmill) seems to be the most beneficial in terms of cardiovascular fitness. Other possibilities you might not have considered are indoor activities such as riding a stationary bike or stair climbing, with or without a ten-pound load to increase the demands on your cardiovascular system. (You need to do a *lot* of ups and downs!)

We hope you're already involved in an active exercise program. But perhaps all this talk about exercise seems tiresome to you. Maybe, in fact, you're like the man who, whenever he had the urge to exercise, would lie down until it passed. However we urge you to give it a try. Plan a program with a friend and be accountable to one another, or enroll in a class, if that will get you started and keep you going. The first few weeks may be hard, but we encourage you to stick with it. We're convinced that it will add life to your years in addition to giving all those benefits to your bones and heart. Moreover, it can help keep you trim. In her practice, Orene has seen women whose mental outlook has improved enormously after they began exercising. It's an antidote for depression.

"But," you may say, "it's so boring!" Then exercise inside, while you watch TV or listen to music. If you have a video cassette recorder, buy an exercise tape and join a filmed class in the privacy of your own home. You can even carry music or inspirational messages outside with you by investing in a tiny radio or cassette player.

As women, we sometimes tend to become such good caretakers of others, that we forget to take care of ourselves. And as Christians, we may feel uncomfortable about putting ourselves first. But when we take preventive measures, we are not being selfish. Prevention is *always* better than the most elaborate of cures. Make it your responsibility to use the information in this chapter to guard yourself against needless expense and distress. Do it for yourself—and for your family.

Chapter Nine

"I'M JUST SO EMOTIONAL!"

The stereotype of the complaining, tearful, impossible-to-get-along-with menopausal female is simply that, a stereotype. Just as no two fingerprints are the same, so no two women will experience an identical passage through menopause. There are as many patterns as there are women on the earth. We want to reemphasize this point before discussing the emotional upheaval, which may or may not accompany menopause.

Some women will move along through the entire climacteric in emotional equilibrium. Many will experience an increased difficulty in coping with frustration or will have greater feelings of stress in situations that were formerly handled with ease. Still there will be no major disruption of their lives. A few, probably no more than fifteen percent, will truly suffer with what one woman called "the crazies," to the point of having difficulty in functioning. They are the exception, not the rule.

If your climacteric is emotionally smooth, we hope this chapter will give you greater empathy with the woman who experiences a more difficult passage. If you should find this a turbulent time, we want to help you understand that you're not alone.

As we've talked with women about the feelings experienced before and during menopause, we found some recurring themes. These are not textbook cases, but are real examples from Orene's practice and from women Bev interviewed. As we examined them, we found they fell into three general categories: loss of control, diminishing self-concept, and the sense that "I'm just not thinking right."

LOSS OF CONTROL

Tearfulness

One distressing facet of loss of control is tearfulness, and it's typified by Chris, a patient whom Orene had seen for some years. She was busy finishing her Ph.D. and managing her family and had always appeared even-tempered and soft-spoken.

Then she came in exclaiming, "I can't imagine what's happening to me. Suddenly—really with practically no reason—I find myself in tears. My mother-in-law didn't specifically compliment me on the cake I'd made for dinner. I cried over that. My husband invited me off on a weekend away from the kids and I began crying as we backed out of the driveway. I watched our youngest walking up the street from school, thought about how big he's getting, and I cried about that. I think I'm keeping the Kleenex company in business this year."

Tearfulness can be precipitated by the simplest situations and quite often a woman is not at all certain why she's so affected. Her family may be shaken by these outbursts, which are not her usual manner. Although the mechanics of this response are not well understood, it is certainly reversible, as the following example illustrates.

Jody, another patient of Orene's, had been taking estrogen for some time and decided to reduce her dosage to .625 of Ogen daily. Within a few weeks, she found she was irritable most of the time. "I felt like crying every day," she explained. "I was just terrible to my husband. I realized after several more weeks that it must be a hormone change, and within four-to-five days of increasing the dose to the old level, I was myself again."

Estrogen can alleviate emotional symptoms. Jody had aggravated her problems by changing the dosage without consulting her doctor. We will discuss the use of estrogen to relieve emotional symptoms in the next chapter.

Free-floating Anxiety or Anger

Other women seem to suffer from what's often referred to as a "free-floating anxiety." It's typified by Janet, a young housewife who helps lead a Bible study. She told Bev, "It's the heebie-jeebies. I feel so on edge. There's just such a sense that all is not quite right. It's nothing specific that I can put my finger on, or analyze, or explain. My husband asks me what triggers it, and I can't tell him. But I never feel completely at ease. The Bible tells us to 'Be anxious for nothing.' But I'm afraid I feel anxious about everything."

Anxiety of nonspecific origin, as Janet describes it, is not unusual, although Orene finds anxiety also may be an exaggerated reaction to particular situations. For instance, a woman may feel frantic because her husband is late getting home from work.

Just as Janet felt anxious about everything, some women feel angry at almost everything. Suddenly small aggravations loom as catastrophes that may lead to emotional explosions. Mary confessed when she entered Orene's office, "I erupt over the slightest little frustration—a child who left books on the kitchen counter when I'm fixing dinner, or my husband forgetting to pick up bread on his way home. My reaction is that *I* don't deserve that kind of treatment, and do I tell them! I know I'm being a witch, but I don't even want to stop. Then I see all the family looking at each other in that funny way."

We will give you some specific handles for controlling your emotions in the next chapter.

Depression

"I'm just so down" is another complaint Orene frequently hears. Often a patient declares, "I don't sleep well at night, and it's such an effort to get up in the morning. I don't really have any purpose."

Depression is one of the most common illnesses in our society. There are large gradations of symptoms, from feeling mildly sad to being painfully ready to give up. We see it at all ages, so depression is certainly not unique to menopause. However, when it occurs at this time of life, it can be a first time event, or it may recur after previous episodes.

A woman may say, "I look around me, and I wonder what I've accomplished, I see myself getting *old* and nothing really gives me any pleasure. It seems like life's basically over for me. Nobody really needs me anymore."

Some women, especially those who experience early menopause and have enjoyed their role as mothers, actually go through a grieving process. They must work through the finality of knowing they'll never have another child, even though logic may tell them that it would be ridiculous to do so at their age. Others begin counting up what they perceive as losses: loss of children (overprotective and overinvolved mothers are particularly prone), loss of purpose, loss of feelings of physical attractiveness, and most particularly, loss of sexuality. A part of us always wants to hold onto what's familiar; when we see it slipping away, we respond with denial, anger, bargaining, and other components of a period of grieving.

A sense of loss may lead to doubting one's self-worth, which one psychologist defines as the root of psychological problems. We need to realize that we have intrinsic value as a child of God, apart from our appearance or our identity as a baby machine. God often has new plans for us once our children are on their own. Women need to establish new goals at this time, whether we focus on a new job or a new project.

Women who are working already have interests outside the home, so they may not be as dependent upon their children and husband. This time of life may also give them new freedom to accept a different kind of job, which may include more travel and/or responsibility than they could handle previously. Many women may be able to travel with their husbands or coordinate their business trips with their spouses so they can work and vacation together. If women look for these new opportunities rather than concentrating on their losses, they are less likely to see midlife as a time of loss.

Another symptom of depression is the sense of failure. Sometimes patients tell Orene, "The things I used to like to do seem worthless and empty. I seem to be losing out."

Orene helps these patients realize that this feeling is a natural part of aging. "How many of your husbands now feel the same way?" she asks. Often women associate feelings with menopause when they are really a part of the midlife crisis, for either a man or a woman. It's natural to evaluate your life once you realize it's half over. As in any critical situation, it's not the crisis that counts, but what you make of it.

If this evaluation can be used positively, a woman might be able to change some attitudes that have led her to make mistakes and learn to capitalize on her strengths. A redirection half way through life is not at all too late to attain success. Look at well-known people who achieved in their later years, such as Grandma Moses, the artist of early Americana and James Michener, the author, who began writing after a severe coronary. An honest evaluation of life often leads women to realize that their lives have not been wasted. The positives do outweigh the negatives. There is, in fact, still much left to be accomplished.

Each of these general symptoms of loss of control—tearfulness, free floating anxiety, and depression—is aggravated by a natural fear, which is followed by an overwhelming sense of panic, and finally, guilt. A woman will often have multiple symptoms of fear, anxiety, anger, and depression, like Terry. "Sometimes I've just gone bananas...blown up and said dreadful things to my husband and my kids. I don't want to do that to them, yet I feel like a smoldering volcano. I'm constantly afraid something will happen to trigger another eruption."

Often women expect themselves to be the perfect wife, mother, and housewife, an expectation which increases their intolerance of themselves and their inability to control their emotions. All of us need to realize that we live in a world which became imperfect when our ancestors, Adam and Eve, disobeyed God. We can't expect perfection, either from ourselves or others or the natural environment around us.

Orene often advises patients to share their emotional difficulties with their families. Instead of trying to be perfect, admit, "I'm feeling—" and ask for understanding. Some patients even tease about their condition, "Beware of mom, she's undergoing 'the change.' " Humor does a lot to help families through tension. It also helps us to take ourselves a little less seriously and to accept ourselves as God's children who are not perfect, who are still under construction. "He's just not finished with me yet." Nor will He be until the day we meet Him in Paradise.

DECLINING SELF-CONCEPT

The second general category of the emotions of menopause is a diminishing self-concept, which is often accompanied by a sense of shame. Trisha, an advertising executive, inevitably experienced hot flushes during an important presentation to a client. "First I'd dab at my upper lip. Then my glasses would start to slide down my nose, and I'd have to take them off to blot the rest of my face. I felt so ashamed to be visibly demonstrating that I was 'a weak female.' Maybe I should have made a joke of it, but I just couldn't. I guess menopause is still something we don't talk about easily."

Ironically, hot flushes often occur at a time when a

woman wants to present herself as an effective female. Since such symptoms simply can't be denied, feelings of anxious anticipation and fear begin to creep in.

Fear

Sometimes women are filled with apprehension as they anticipate menopause. "I didn't know what to expect," Ruth said. "My mother died when I was ten, and my grandmother raised me," she continued, explaining that she felt totally unprepared when she began throwing off the covers in the middle of the night and realized she might be starting menopause.

"I was afraid of being a physical and emotional wreck," she admitted to Orene. "Also, I was afraid of being old, of losing my attractiveness. I immediately had visions of myself with a big black moustache, and I was afraid that my husband wouldn't love me anymore, that he might even start looking for a younger woman."

All of Ruth's fears seemed to converge on "what ifs'?" and were not truly realistic. If Ruth had begun preparing for menopause when she became thirty-five, she would have avoided many of these fears. If you are feeling fearful, ask yourself, "How many of my fears are 'what ifs'?" Then remember the biblical principle: "Do not worry about tomorrow, for tomorrow will worry about its own things. Sufficient for the day is its own trouble" (Matt. 6:34).

Ruth's preoccupation with her appearance is a widespread concern during menopause. In fact, some of the same feelings that occurred in adolescence, when we coped with acne and awkwardness, may surface once again in exaggerated feelings of ugliness.

Sue confessed to Bev, "I'd always thought I looked pretty good for my age. Then my husband and I decided to have our picture taken for our twenty-fifth anniversary. My husband looked just great in every picture. And there wasn't one of me I could bear. Who was that old lady with the sagging eyelids and those deep, deep lines around her mouth? What a moment of truth!"

Sue spoke, too, of finding she could no longer thread a needle and realizing she needed bifocals. Such concrete symptoms of old age are particularly threatening because they can't be easily denied, and we are reminded of them every time we look up a telephone number or try to read a road map.

Sue continued, "The trauma of getting glasses was bad enough, but when I got them and could really see, I could also see all these wrinkles. I didn't look nearly as great as I'd thought I did. I'd have traded the glasses back in, but my arms weren't long enough to read the newspaper or a phone book."

Bev remembers her own mother's distress after surgical menopause. A lovely picture of her mother at about age thirty-five had always stood on her father's desk. Suddenly, it was gone. Bev's aunt told her later that her mother thought she had aged terribly and just couldn't bear what she considered the difference between the then and the now.

It's unfortunate that society has laid on us the feeling that older is ugly, or that sexiness and beauty are a woman's greatest assets. Actress Evelyn Keyes, who now plays "more mature roles," fights to overcome the myth that beauty and youth are essential. "[Because of] all this concentrated effort given to preserving one particular time slot in our life spans, we are missing out on what might very well be the best interlude of all."

She suggests that perhaps women need a cream that will enhance "every new and lovely wrinkle...Wouldn't it be nice to have something to look forward to (Oh happy day! I'm going gray!), instead of spending your young years worrying and trying to avoid that which is inevitable to us all?"[1]

Feelings that lower self-concept can also sometimes leave us with a real sense of loneliness. Here's how Karen expressed it. "Sometimes I feel like I'm the only one who feels as I do. All the women in my Bible study are younger. My husband doesn't really understand what I'm going through. And my kids aren't capable of thinking about anything but themselves. I don't feel so terrible that I need medication. And I suppose I should try to get out and meet new people, but it just seems too much effort. I feel bad about myself, and I just can't share that with other people."

Indeed, menopause is, for many women, a lonely event. Often our parents are no longer vigorous enough to help. Children are far too preoccupied with getting on with the business of their lives to be either sympathetic or attentive. And talking with others may seem socially unacceptable to us.

For women who are not married, menopause may bring a particular sense of loneliness, as well as frustration and sadness. To them, there is an aching finality about it. Here is concrete evidence that they will never bear children; a goal they may not have allowed themselves to dwell on previously will never be reached. Their feelings may culminate in what one single woman described as "a time of grieving, accompanied by a sense of uselessness and inadequacy." She added, "I think I could write a chapter for you on the feelings of never carrying out what nature intended me to do."

These feelings are appropriate at this age, and need to be faced so that each woman can work toward a new equilibrium of adjustment and acceptance.

I'M JUST NOT THINKING RIGHT

The final general symptom of menopause is the feeling of a loss of mental acuity. Although the hot flush has been diagnosed as a response to brain mechanisms during menopause, no one has yet defined well the change in thought mechanisms which also can occur. Over and over Orene's patients report a loss of concentration, perhaps accompanied by hot flushes.

Lack of Concentration

"I'm really frightened at the way I can't seem to keep focused on a subject," Betty stated. "I start to read the newspaper and find my mind wandering. It even happens when I'm reading the Bible. I finish a chapter, and I've no idea what it says."

Betty added that she's been thinking about taking classes to get her realtor's license. "It seems so difficult to study. I don't know if I can handle it, especially when my memory doesn't seem to be nearly as sharp as it used to be. Frankly, I'm beginning to wonder if I'm getting senile."

It's normal for Betty to wonder if her forgetfulness is the beginning of senility, early Alzheimer's, or just a downward trend in her productivity that will never reverse itself. A loss of memory could even be a symptom of an organic brain disease. The chances are most likely, however, that this is a temporary menopausal symptom, which will disappear when the hot flushes and other symptoms subside.

Confusion

Another mental symptom that distresses many patients is a sense of confusion in handling situations in their lives. At times, it's particularly hard for them to separate what is a normal reaction to circumstances and what may be overreacting.

For instance, on Monday Terry's father called to tell her that her mother, diagnosed ten years previously as manic-depressive, was in the hospital in intensive care after suffering a heart attack.

Tuesday she learned that her father's favorite sister had died. Then, just as she prepared to meet her father at the funeral and fly north with him to be with her mother, her oldest son "dropped by to talk." Terry was shocked to hear that he and his wife had agreed to separate.

"It was all I could do to keep from bawling right on the spot," she later told Orene. "But that would be just so—so menopausal!"

"Wouldn't you have been upset over these things ten years ago, too?" Orene asked.

"Oh! Well, yeah, I see," Terry replied with relief, as she realized that her response was appropriate to the circumstances, rather than the overreaction of a menopausal female.

A mental symptom that often is specific to menopause, however, is the great difficulty some women suddenly experience in getting organized. Anne told how she'd finish breakfast in the morning and think, *I really should put the dishes in the dishwasher.* Then she'd decide to do it later. She'd tell herself, *Now I'll make the beds. Well, I will. Later.*

She reported, "I'd lie down on the couch or watch TV. Then I'd get down on myself for wasting time, and I'd go through this hysterical five o'clock scramble to do everything I should have done earlier. Dinner guests were more than I could cope with."

One of the most deceptive aspects of emotional upheaval during natural menopause is that these symptoms may occur before a woman experiences many physical manifestations. Unable to pinpoint a cause, she begins to wonder if she's going "round the bend."

This was true of Anne, who, at fifty-two, had noticed almost no changes in her periods when her feelings of confusion began. She was further plagued by a "terrible insecurity. I withdrew from others, did anything I could to avoid being with people. I cried easily over the most innocent remarks, often reading negative things into them. Church was agony because I felt I had to pretend I was normal and smile as though nothing was wrong."

Her own physician failed to recognize the root of her problem, and she was convinced that "if this kept up, I'd be committed." It was only when she saw a psychiatrist who ordered an FSH test and found a low estrogen level that she was able to receive help.

For most women, the emotional upheavals of menopause come and go. There are good times interspersed with the not-so-wonderful.

The big question always arises: *why* do we feel like this? Are these feelings a reflection of the attitudes of our society and the people around us? Are they caused by the life circumstances in which we find ourselves? Do they stem from our own psychological makeup? Or are they rooted in the physical changes of menopause?

All of these factors are so intertwined that it's often difficult for a physician to evaluate. In a later chapter, we'll examine the effect of attitudes on our experience. But now let's explore the other causes.

ROOTS OF MENOPAUSAL EMOTIONS

Social, Circumstantial

To put it mildly, the timing of menopause certainly leaves a lot to be desired! It arrives at a point in our lives when a host of changes all converge. These may confuse the issue and make it difficult to sort out cause and effect. For instance, if we are career women, we reach menopause at a time when we're being pressured by the younger "rising stars" of our field. And if we want a new career, we may find that most companies are wary of someone they'll have to plug into retirement benefits in a comparatively short time.

If we have children, we may hit menopause just as we learn the validity of the old saying, "Little children, little problems. Big children, big problems." The teen years are notoriously a time of trauma. And later, many of us find that our homes seem to be equipped with revolving doors, through which our grown offspring come and go. Or perhaps menopause comes as we cope with the vacuum that remains after our children cut their parental cords.

At the same time, our aging parents need more and more of our time and energy. "You didn't call me yesterday," or "Can you drive me to the dentist/store/hairdresser/doctor?" become familiar refrains. We find ourselves the "sandwich" generation, squeezed between the old and the young. Just as we're coping with a son who wants to move into his girlfriend's apartment, we may get a call that our dad's suffered a stroke.

Moreover, menopause and midlife crisis, though they are not the same thing, may come at the same time, or they may overlap. Menopause may well coincide with the "I guess I'll never" blues of middle age, or "middlescence," as one writer calls it. ("Guess I'll never write the great American novel." "Guess I'll never be president of the company." "Guess I'll never win the club championship.") A wife in menopause and a husband in mid-life crisis, as we've noted, are not the stuff of which marvelous marriages are made!

Another difficulty is the changing role of women today. As one fifty-year-old woman expressed it, "I don't know whether I'm supposed to be starting a new career or baking cookies for my grandson."

The most confused and depressed reactions at midlife for men and women, states G. Mitchell in *Human Sex Difference: A Primatologist's Perspective,* come to those in the social transition group. Both completely "traditional" women and men and "liberated" women and men handle times of change better than "transitional" women who are no longer fulfilling the mother role, but lack the skills for the "liberated" role.[2]

Psychological

Some doctors have dismissed the emotional upheaval of menopause by patly stating that psychological problems during menopause are simply extensions of previously existing disorders. The woman who experienced exaggerated fears in the past, for instance, will have new fears during menopause.

Others say it is a mind-set, based upon expectations a woman develops, which are in turn based on observations of other members of her family. ("Mother had a tough time, and so will I.") Still others say a woman's emotional reaction depends upon her basic personality. Is she an optimist who tends to see the best in situations and to look forward to a better tomorrow, rather than dwelling on the past or the present? Or is she naturally melancholic, a "woe is me" personality, or what one husband described as "a Pollyanna in reverse"? Typifying this difference is an overheard conversation:

"I'm forty today, and my life is half over."

"I just had my fortieth birthday, and I figure I have half my life yet to live!"

Some women displace their fears and feelings into physical complaints. These are more socially acceptable and will bring attention from others. They may take the form of headaches, gastrointestinal distress, "back problems."

This was the case with Louise, who had retired a year earlier as a highly successful shoe clerk and came to Orene with menopausal symptoms, plus nausea and vomiting, which are not usually related to menopause. Orene altered Louise's estrogens until she had good control of the hot flashes. But the nausea and vomiting persisted. She then sent Louise to one psychiatrist who felt she had no problem. So Orene ordered a full gastrointestinal workup, and no abnormality was found. Now it was important to reassure Louise and to convince her that she did not have a serious physical disease and that these were not hormonal symptoms. But despair, with frequent bouts of tearfulness, accentuated her other symptoms. Finally, she saw another psychiatrist who began her on an antidepressant. It was almost a year before she began "acting like Louise" again.

It takes a sensitive physician or team of physicians to screen other causes for symptoms like this and to couple appropriate medication with short-term supportive psychotherapy. But when they do, many symptoms often disappear.

Physical

Can emotional distress be rooted specifically in the falling estrogen levels? There are few well-controlled reports to answer this question. The relationship between hormone balance and emotional response in the postpartum period (after giving birth) and also in PMS is fairly well established. It would seem logical that diminishing estrogen would affect the nervous system and women's emotional well-being at menopause. Still, some doctors say that a caring relationship with the patient is more important than the dispensing of medication.

Many patients, however, insist that their experience indicates a definite relationship between hormone level and emotional well-being, since estrogen replacement therapy brings them such dramatic relief. There is no question for a patient named Anne that her ability to concentrate and feel in control of herself improved quickly after beginning estrogen replacement therapy. Another patient Nancy had a tremendous sleep disturbance with chronic fatigue. She didn't deal with small stresses well until she started estrogen and stopped waking with hot flashes four and five times each night.

On the other hand, Sara tried various doses of hormones and still felt unable to eat, sleep, and function well in her job. After finding that her estrogen dose had adequately reduced her FSH level, she was also placed on an antidepressant. Within several weeks, her entire sense of well-being improved and she could again function at her necessary level of responsibility.

Many of Orene's patients have improved with the administration of hormones, which makes a fairly strong case for the emotional effects of estrogen deprivation. There is an intricate balance in some women that we hope in years to come will be understood and defined in such a way that we will know why certain physical and emotional symptoms do respond to estrogen. We'll look in more detail at hormone therapy, and many other avenues of dealing with your emotions, in the next chapter.

Chapter Ten

COPING WITH YOUR EMOTIONS

The first thing most menopausal women think about when their emotions surge out of hand is that they need hormones. Surely, they believe, there will be a magic cure-all for depression, confusion, anxiety, for any of their consuming feelings.

However, estrogen therapy for these symptoms is not always either necessary or advisable. How, then, should you deal with your emotions?

Your Doctor's Help

When emotions go on the rampage, it's often difficult for a doctor to decide whether to confront the problem from a medical or psychological standpoint. The two are delicately intertwined, and doctors still don't fully understand the relationship between hormone deficiency and the symptoms we discussed in the last chapter. The first approach many take today is to check the FSH to see if it's elevated, which would indicate that the estrogen level is low. If it is, and symptoms either develop during the climacteric or are aggravated by it, then they prescribe hormonal therapy to see if it helps. Possibly they'll also suggest counseling, depending upon the patient's circumstances and history.

Jane was just twenty-seven when she had a hysterectomy with only a small portion of the ovary left in place. There was enough ovarian tissue to provide normal hormone output until her early forties, when she began taking 1.25 milligrams of Premarin a day. She experienced some swelling in her feet, and on her own, decreased her dosage to a third of what had been prescribed.

Soon hospitalized with a combination of symptoms including trembling inside, no energy, and a fear that she would lose control, she declared, "I feel I'm on the doorstep of a nervous breakdown." Her doctor wasn't sure if these symptoms stemmed from outside events or hormone deficiency. (We still don't understand the intricate mechanisms of brain and body interactions.) But since she insisted, "There's really no problem in my life that should make me so disturbed," a serum FSH was ordered and showed marked elevation, indicating menopausal estrogen deprivation. She was placed on 2.5 milligrams of estrogen per day and asked not to change the medication without calling her doctor. In two weeks, her "nervous breakdown" symptoms subsided.

It's important to understand, though, that there is no evidence to justify the use of estrogens in the treatment of primary psychological problems, that is, those which existed before menopause. Surveys show no consistent associations between moods, or psychological state, and estrogen deprivation.

For some women, drugs such as tranquilizers or mood elevators may give relief and be appropriate for short term use. Using them to get you over the hump is not giving up but sensibly accepting available help. Mood elevators, or antidepressants, are usually better than tranquilizers since there seems to be more depression than anxiety in menopause. If there is a combination of depression and anxiety, mood elevators often will give both a sedative and an antidepressive action.

Remember, too, tranquilizers such as Valium and Tranxene do create some body dependency after a while, while the tricyclic antidepressants such as Elavil are not habit-forming. After a period of treatment, most patients reach a point when they don't need these medications anymore. They forget to take them and begin to feel like themselves again. Sometimes, however, it's best to step down the dosage gradually, rather than to stop abruptly.

Mary, a nursing instructor, knew she was at high risk for uterine cancer if she took estrogen, but she came to Orene complaining of being so emotional at times that she felt almost "out of control." In addition, hot flushes awakened her four to five times a night.

There were two alternatives. Mary could begin on estrogen and progesterone, as long as Orene took endometrial biopsies every so often to be sure Mary didn't develop cancer. This measure would probably control the hot flushes and fatigue. But Mary had been on an antidepressant in the past for mild depression, and she admitted, "I feel a lot like I did that other time." So the second alternative was to take an antidepressant at bedtime to try to better the sleep pattern and, it was hoped, to improve the depression.

"The hot flushes are a nuisance," Mary admitted, "but what really bothers me are the feelings of loss of control."

Since Mary had a stable marriage and wasn't going through any obvious situational changes, Orene chose to start Mary on an antidepressant. Although the dosage was small, Mary was able to perform well at work and at home again.

If your physician feels that drug therapy is indicated, then you may begin on estrogens or other medications that may improve your symptoms. The importance of your being "tuned-in" to your body changes cannot be overemphasized, and it is your responsibility to convey these changes in your emotions to your doctor.

If drug therapy doesn't seem appropriate to you or your physician, by all means seek counseling to deal with these symptoms.

Counseling

You may be one of the fortunate women who live in an area where specific counseling is available in a clinic or women's health center to give you support and to help answer your emotional needs during menopause. Or, if you feel menopause has intensified a previously existing difficulty, and if you sense that it's not responding to medical treatment, you may want to seek the help of a trained counselor on the staff of a large church or perhaps a psychologist or psychiatrist. Do be sure, however, that you find one who is specifically equipped to deal with women's midlife wellness. Your physician or perhaps your clergy can lead you to the appropriate person.

Psychologists agree that menopause often coincides with the well-defined empty nest syndrome. These feelings may be eased by creating new interests and new avenues for expression. At times, it can require supportive therapy, as in Marcia's case. She was highly involved in her children's high school activities, rooting at swim meets, helping with the school operetta, serving on the PTA. Her husband had encouraged her to be active but preferred to spend his own free time reading or listening to his stereo.

Marcia's uterus and ovaries were removed during the winter, and she was not given hormone therapy because of fibrocystic breast disease. By the time her youngest child was packing for college, she began to feel panicky whenever she was alone at home. She was all right when someone else was there, but she found it unbearable to be in the house by herself. Was the cause hormonal or emotional?

It was only when Marcia began therapy that she realized her panic stemmed from watching her last child leave home and from her concern that she and her husband no longer had anything in common. After a few sessions, she could be alone in the house without feeling distraught. A year later, she reported that her marriage was better than it had ever been.

What Are Friends For?

Your best human resource during menopause may well be friends who are your age or older. They have either "been there", or "are there," and together you can enjoy a foxhole-buddy camaraderie. You can laugh at the ridiculousness of your symptoms and at yourselves. You can gently tease and be teased by such remarks as, "Is it hot in here?"

Who but a good friend can reassure you of her affection when, that very morning, you've been less than lovable with your family? As teenagers, some of us thought our mothers were just "too sickening" when they embraced their friends. Now we see clearly that their friends may have been the only people in their lives who would really listen to them and understand their problems.

It's unfortunate to see relationships like Eileen and Barb's. Recently Eileen remarked to Barb, "You've changed a lot. You're much nicer than when our boys were in high school together."

Barb suddenly realized that her "not nice" phase coincided with her menopausal years. Why had she never mentioned her difficulties to Eileen? How different their relationship might have been if she'd been able to discuss her feelings with her friend.

Perhaps you are a private person and feel reluctant to "dump" on others. But if you'll be open with another woman, you may give her an opportunity to share with you. You'll both gain immeasurably.

Networking

Networking is an extension of such sharing with your friends. It's a gathering together of women who are in a common situation, the climacteric, both to share and to learn from experts.

The Center for Climacteric Studies in Gainesville, Florida, has begun groups in various parts of the state, which now are spreading to other parts of the country, from Kansas to California to Connecticut, and even to Australia. They're called "CLOUT," for CLimacteric OUTreach. Their objective is to provide the information and feedback that will assure optimal health in midlife. They accomplish this by asking women what they want, then presenting midlife wellness seminars and workshops, which both answer their needs and give them a chance to share with one another. A similar organization, VIDO, Women in Menopause, reaches out through trained leaders to 160 chapters in the Netherlands.

In addition, some women's clinics in various parts of our country give women a chance to exchange here's-what-works-for-me ideas and to learn together about various facets of menopausal management. When the menopause clinic in Santa Monica, California, was featured on TV, coordinator Ellen Neiman remarked, "The walls haven't stopped reverberating, the need is so great."

One study of climacteric women indicated that their sense of well-being didn't improve while taking any specific hormone or tranquilizer. But those who went to see a health care worker benefited through avenues of open communication. The need seems clear, and we look forward to new avenues which will evolve throughout the country. Perhaps you'd like to start one in your church or community. The study guide at the end of this book is specially designed for group activities. (For information, you might want to write The Center for Climacteric Studies, University of Florida, 901 N.W. 8th Ave., Suite B1, Gainesville, FL 32601.)

Your Family

Even if our mothers suffered in silence during menopause, we don't have to. "Menopause" is at last a word that can be spoken, and we feel it's much healthier for the entire family if they understand something of what's happening to you. Of course, neither long "organ recitals" nor the belief that you have a license to behave abominably will help to enhance family relationships. It does mean explaining what you're feeling and why you might act a little "off-the-wall" from time to time. It also means assuring your family that "this too shall pass."

One woman alerted her family to her mood swings by posting a sign she found in a stationery store on the home bulletin board. It warned, "My pleasing disposition is subject to change without notice." Another found a sign shaped in the form of a dial, with a pointer which could be aimed at such mood indicators as "Coast clear," "Proceed with caution," and "Danger! Explosives!"

No matter how much you try to communicate, don't expect a lot of support from teenagers or offspring who are busy finishing school, paying for their cars, starting careers, or setting up households. But do seek your husband's support and forbearance. One wife recalls with infinite gratitude how her sensitive husband learned to read her moods and sometimes put his arms around her and said, "It's OK. Go ahead and cry."

Surely, such a man is worth his weight in gold. But remember, not all men are so discerning. So tell your husband what you feel and need; don't expect him to be a mind reader. One woman did just this during a Marriage Encounter, a weekend retreat for married couples. It gave her the opportunity to write to him, "If I react in what seems an unreasonable way, please don't just abandon me and say to yourself, 'It's the menopause.' What seems unreasonable to you is very real to me, and I need you to help me work through these feelings."

Another approach, when you feel angry or contentious and are tempted to direct those feelings toward your husband, is simply to say to him, "I really need a hug." Few men can resist. Hugs are terrific therapy for you both!

Help Yourself

At a time of life when you may feel helpless, there are things you can do for yourself. Some of them may seem obvious, but have you tried any of them? You may be surprised at how effective they can be.

l. Do everything you can to look your best.

It's a fact that the better you look, the better you feel. So take the time to find a new, becoming hairstyle. If you've never spent time learning to apply makeup, perhaps you'll want to investigate how the skillful use of a light foundation, creamy blush, and a little eye makeup can enhance your appearance.

You might also want to have a color analysis, so you know which shades make your skin look clear, your hair shiny, your eyes sparkling. By all means learn all you can about your most becoming lines and styles in clothes. (A book such as *Uniquely You,* by Betty Nethery and Beverly Bush Smith, which deals with both inner and outer beauty, might be helpful to you.) Then, put on a dress or blouse or sweater you love. It's amazing how much better you'll feel and how much positive feedback you'll receive from others. People are naturally attracted to those who look attractive.

2. Exercise.

Not only is exercise excellent for your bones and your heart, it's terrific psychological therapy. Many of Orene's patients tell of the "high" they experience when running, or the "cleansing" they feel after twenty or thirty minutes of swimming, or the invigorating effect of aerobic dancing. Choose something you enjoy. You'll be amazed how it will enhance your ability to cope and your sense of well-being.

3. Try compartmentalizing your life.

A doctor told us recently that she began feeling frustrated because she needed to stay home with her baby instead of continuing to play tennis in the evening. "But whenever I feel thwarted, I compartmentalize it. I tell myself that there's going to be a time when I'll play tennis again. Certain activities or accomplishments are appropriate for different times of my life. My advice is: Don't resent not being able to do a certain thing. Be glad you used to enjoy that activity and will enjoy it again, some day in the future."

Her observations seem to echo Ecclesiastes: "To everything there is a season, A time for every purpose under heaven: A time to be born, And a time to die: A time to plant, And a time to pluck what is planted" (Ecc. 3:1).

The woman who learns to accept the rhythm of the changes of her life is well on her way to mental wellness.

4. "Don't let the sun go down on your anger."

Anger, when internalized, can become depression. So if you're "ready to explode," it's all right to express your anger, so long as you don't allow it to tear down relationships. Perhaps you can express it in a hard game of tennis or by jogging or even making bread. "Mad bread" is the best, you know, because it's so thoroughly kneaded.

Perhaps your anger needs to be stated verbally in an "I" statement. This expression of feeling in the first person helps defuse your emotion by allowing you to be honest about your feelings, yet it doesn't foster hostility. For example, "I feel so angry when—," as opposed to "you" accusations, "You always forget to—."

If you find yourself directing your anger at an innocent party, two words are vital: "I'm sorry."

5. Do something for someone else.

Introspection is fine, unless it gets out of hand and begins to slide into self-pity which, as we saw in the last chapter, inevitably leads to depression. You can either continue down the tube or take charge of those feelings and begin to look outward.

There's always a friend or neighbor who needs your care or attention. Make a phone call. Take a neighbor shopping or to lunch. Bring in dinner for someone who's ill. The needs are great, the helpers few.

As you can see, different solutions work for different

people. If you're experiencing emotional difficulties at this time, don't give up and don't assume that no one understands or that nothing can be done. Today, there are more avenues of help open than ever before. Look over the various possibilities we've given you for coping, and make a change for the better today.

Chapter Eleven

THE SHAPING OF ATTITUDES

The advertising slogan, "You've come a long way, baby!" might well be applied to recent advances in dealing with menopause. Once the presence or absence of menopausal symptoms was considered simply a matter of the woman's attitude. Some doctors thought those who suffered programmed themselves to think: *It's a dreadful time, and I'm going to suffer.* Even women doctors thought hot flashes were "all in a woman's mind."

Still, there's no doubt that our experience with menopause is affected by attitudes, both those of our culture and of the significant people in our lives. In order to liberate ourselves from old tapes playing in our subconscious minds, let's look at the attitude of other cultures and then at our own to see how mindsets and physical responses can be conditioned by society. We'll also see which attitudes are rational and which are just myths and old wives' tales.

OTHER CULTURES

To understand attitudes toward menopause in other times and other places, we must first consider outlooks on menstruation.

Remember how a woman's menstrual period was called her "uncleanness" in biblical times. Listen to some of the laws from Leviticus.

"If a woman has a discharge, and the discharge from her body is blood, she shall be set apart seven days; and whoever touches her shall be unclean until evening.

"Everything that she lies on during her impurity shall be unclean; also everything that she sits on shall be unclean.

"Whoever touches her bed shall wash his clothes, and bathe in water, and be unclean until evening" (Lev. 15: 19-21).

"If any man lies with her at all, so that her impurity is on him, he shall be unclean seven days; and every bed on which he lies shall be unclean" (Lev. 15:24).

This sounds more like the old-fashioned health regulations for leprosy than for a natural physical condition, but that's not all. Once a woman's discharge ceased, she had to count seven days before she was considered clean. On the eighth day, she took two turtledoves or young pigeons to the priest, who offered one for a sin offering and the other for a burnt offering, making "atonement for her before the Lord for her unclean discharge."

A woman was virtually in isolation for two weeks out of every month. She couldn't even go to the temple. Although childbearing was extremely important in that society, surely she experienced a sense of release when she stopped menstruating and became free of all these restrictions.

Even in many cultures today, women have greater freedom and status after menopause. In parts of Africa and in Bali, the postmenopausal woman and the virgin girl work together at ceremonies from which women of child-bearing age are barred.

In Rajput, India, younger women must be veiled, and while menstruating, they're considered "dangerous" and "defiling" and are separated from men.

Not surprisingly, a survey of these women showed they were eager to become postmenopausal and pleased to be growing older. After they stopped menstruating, they could remove their veils and talk with men. They could have input in decision-making related to farming and could mingle and talk and socialize with the men. In short, they could do all the things that were forbidden while they were menstruating. Interestingly, none of the five hundred Rajput women personally interviewed during their climacteric by anthropologist

Marcha Flint reported any negative symptoms.

In *A Time to Reap,* Nancy Aron and associates studied five different subcultures and found marked differences in their views of menopause. Middle Europeans saw a possible decline in emotional health. The Turks, Persians, and North Africans were worried about a decline in physical health. However the Arabs welcomed the end to ritual uncleanliness, for the menstrual taboos spelled out in Leviticus are repeated in the Koran. Contact with a menstruating woman is forbidden; and after menstruation, the woman must perform a ritual purification of her body. Muslim taboos extend to a prohibition on prayer, fasting, contact with the Koran, or any other religious act.

Nancy Aron's conclusion is that women's responses to menopause and middle age are shaped by the culture in which they grow up. What they see as gains and losses is a product of earlier life experiences and the resulting resources a woman brings to middle age, as well as the dominant values in her culture.

Remember, too, that not all societies place such emphasis on youth and youthfulness as we do. Among the Navajo Indians, for instance, women maintain a high position in the society throughout life. And according to Estelle Fuchs' book, *The Second Season,* they report no menopausal difficulties.

Another study of the Navajos, reported by Ann Wright, indicates that very few of the women had ever discussed this event with anyone. There was, in fact, no Navajo word for menopause. (In contrast, the word used to describe menopause in New Guinea means "she can do nothing more.")

One Navajo woman's outlook was, "It just happens that we were made like that. You have children, then you stop. You get periods to have babies and there are no more periods after you stop having babies." Menopause brought no change in status; a woman's normal productive and domestic activities were unaffected by this change. Thus they regard menopause simply as a part of the life cycle, marking the transition from the reproductive years to the valued stage of old age.

In many cultures, to become a grandparent is to reach a highpoint in life. In China elders have always been revered; today they are a necessary part of the household, since it is the grandparents who provide child care while parents go out to work.

In her examination of the status of menopausal and postmenopausal women in thirty different cultures, Pauline Bart found that in only two did women's status decrease after menopause. In those two societies, on the Trobriand Islands and the Marquesas, there were no close grandparent-grandchild relationships.

Around the world in other cultures, women's attitudes toward menopause seem to be shaped by their society, falling into two vastly different general categories: "loss of" or "freedom from," as described by Brian M. DuToit, Ph.D., professor of anthropology at the University of Florida.

OUR CHANGING ATTITUDES

In our culture what are the dominant attitudes which strongly affect our reactions to menopause?

Accent on Youth

Our society reveres youth and places great emphasis upon acting and looking young. The supreme compliment is, "You can't be that old! You look much younger!" Or, "Surely you're not a grandmother!" Notice all the ads for everything from hair coloring to plastic surgery that appeal to this desire.

For many, menopause is synonymous with growing old. In the "All in the Family" menopause episode, Edith's first reaction to her daughter's suggestion that she might be menopausal is, "Oh my! At my age? Oh, no, I ain't supposed to change yet....Now I'm gonna be an old lady!"

Later, she's temporarily consoled by the thought of someday having grandchildren, until she realizes that would make her a grandmother.

Even before women become "old ladies," they're the victims of a number of stereotypes that focus on middle age. All too often they're cast as over-the-hill or useless females, argumentative mothers-in-law, or wicked stepmothers.

The more a woman accepts these stereotypes, the more likely she is to report feelings of despair, a sense of having no positive purpose. Depression, in such cases, is probably not due to hormonal changes, but to a loss of self-esteem, as G. Mitchell points out in *Human Sex Difference: A Primatologist's Perspective.*

Estelle Fuchs in *The Second Season,* says, "So many women have been raised, unrealistically for the modern world, to identify their personal worth almost exclusively with their looks, their beauty. Such women are, unless life develops a new resiliency, to suffer great trauma with aging."[1]

Sociologist Ernest Becker, critiquing Sigmund Freud's psychoanalytic interpretation of menopause difficulties, also points to social conditioning. "We create menopausal depression in women by not seeing to it that women in their forties are armed with more than one justification for their lives."[2]

Moreover, some feel that our culture confronts women with a self-fulfilling prophecy that they will experience midlife emotional breakdown. Observes Estelle Fuchs, "It takes a lot of courage and strength to withstand the withering effects of a rejecting world."[3]

The Silent Treatment

Partly because of these negative attitudes toward this stage of life, and partly because of a holdover of the Victorian taboos against talking about "female problems," we've also suffered from a we-don't-talk-about-it syndrome. "Menopause" was a word to be whispered. In the "All in the Family" program, Archie's daughter uses the word during a conversation in a coffee shop. Archie immediately shushes her, looking around in embarrassment to see who may have heard. Similarly, after her discussion of menopause with her daughter, Edith insists, "There's your father. Don't you say a word to him about this!"

Menopause simply wasn't talked about in polite society. Often women couldn't discuss it with their husbands or even any but the very best of friends. Many women today are not aware of their mothers' experience with menopause, because not a word was said.

Some of us remember when menstruation was also hush-hush. Heaven forbid that your date should know it was "that time." Certainly, that's changed. Today, we may see a young man obligingly carrying his date's tampons in his backpack when they go biking. Another boyfriend talks freely about how change of diet helped his girl's premenstrual syndrome.

Today we're also making progress in bringing menopause out of the closet. But many people still have a long way to go toward being open, honest, and at ease with the subject.

Male Attitudes

Sometimes men can be worse than women in fostering negative outlooks. An eighty-year-old father confronted his daughter with, "Well, now you're getting to that age, aren't you? You know, the change. Well, I hope you're not going to be like your mother! She was so depressed. I'd tell her to go out and buy a new dress. And she'd say, 'I don't want a new dress!' She was impossible!"

Fortunately, the daughter, remembering that her mother had undergone surgical menopause without hormone therapy, refused to expect that she, too, would be "impossible."

Similarly, a minister counseling a widower who contemplated marrying a younger woman, cautioned, "Are you sure you want to go through the trauma of menopause again?" We're happy to report that the widower's love was much greater than his concern over this impending "trauma."

Certainly a husband's attitude can make an enormous difference in a woman's perception of herself at this time. Many physicians find two extremes. There's the husband who is staunchly supportive and may be the first to suggest that his wife come in for an office visit.

"You know," one husband said, "I'm having trouble living with these feelings you're having. Make an appointment with your doctor and see if there's anything you can do about it." Another such husband actually pointed out to his wife what was happening before she realized it. "Have you noticed, you're not yourself lately?" he said.

Then there is that rarity, the husband who doesn't want to have anything to do with it. "It's *your* problem," he shrugs and may even react by simply moving out. But almost always this happens because *two* people are in a time of transition: the menopausal female and the mid-life male. When these passages coincide, the husband has great difficulty being supportive.

Then consider the naturally impatient man who tries his best. In "All in the Family," Archie *tried* to be patient, kind, and agreeable, as the doctor suggested. But enough was enough. At last he erupted with, "I know all about your woman's troubles there, Edith, but when I had the hernia, I didn't make you wear the truss!"

Other men simply don't know how to give meaningful encouragement. The husband who wanted his wife to buy a new dress was trying to help, though obviously a new dress didn't meet his wife's needs. Another man encouraged his wife to take a trip to Europe with her best friend. "Don't worry, we can get along just fine without you," he urged, thinking to release her to enjoy herself. Instead, her reaction was, "Nobody needs me anymore."

Communication is *so* important and will help you avoid the trap of, "But I thought you..." or "Can't you *see* that...?"

Doctors' Outlook

Gradually, we're emerging from an age when doctors regarded menopause as a purely physical phenomenon and failed to focus on the total person in dealing with the symptoms. We can all sing the Doxology over that.

However, we can sympathize with the physician when a patient comes in with a dozen subjective complaints, expecting her doctor to sort them all out. Is this a medical problem or an emotional problem? It can be tough for the doctor to determine. Of course, we all long for more physicians who are sympathetic and empathetic, but this may not be as simple as it sounds. We are just in the pioneering phase of correlating the brain, emotions, hormones, and all the other components of this complex process.

The Feminist Influence

Dr. James Dobson, in his radio broadcasts on menopause, has decried the damage done by some feminists who, in their effort to prove that women can do anything men can do, deny the fact of menopause. They would have us believe that neither menopause nor the menstrual cycle affects women and their abilities or performance. Thus women who *do* find themselves affected feel abnormal and guilty.

However, most physicians will tell you that there frequently *is* a difference between the response of the housewife and the working woman. The woman who is career-oriented is usually not as introspective as the woman who does not have a career or a specific area of interest outside the home. The person who looks outward is less likely to be bothered by her menstrual periods and is less prone to bring problems of menopause to her doctor's attention.

Interestingly, in one study of different cultures, the balance of joy and sorrow for menopausal women was most positive for the Central Europeans and the Arabs.

Psychological well-being was lowest among the Persian women, who represent the midpoint between tradition and modernity. It seemed that the most important factor in attitude and adaptation to life change was the stability of the women's position, not the position itself.

Perhaps, then, the introspective woman of today feels herself caught somewhere between tradition and modernity. The world gives her disquieting messages that the traditional mother/grandmother role is not enough. But the other extreme, getting a job, looks terrifying and impossible at her age.

Women who are committed Christians have a rock upon which to base their stability, their love of the Lord and the guidance of His Word in the Bible. Often these women check changing values against Scripture, pray, and then decide what is God's will for their lives.

Pat, after a period of study and prayer, took a part-time bookkeeping job, which allows her to continue teaching a weekly Bible study and to baby-sit occasionally for her grandson. Jackie, on the other hand, realized that she and her husband did not need the extra income, so she did not look for employment. Instead she began visiting patients in convalescent homes as a volunteer ministry.

As Christians we can overcome many of the emotional symptoms of menopause once we realize that our secular society often gives us destructive messages. Also, advertising and television sitcoms and soaps can mislead us by directly and indirectly making us believe that we should always be comfortable. Got a backache? Take this medication. Indigestion? Quick relief with Tums for the tummy. Too warm and hot this summer? Cool off with a refreshing drink of—.

One menopausal woman spent much of her time after

her children left home watching the soaps. She was timid in social situations because of her hearing problem and the hearing aid she wore, so she had never been active in her church or local clubs. Day after day, she watched programs where the husband was engaged in extramarital affairs.

Soon she began suspecting that her husband (a very loyal and mild-mannered man) was involved with other women, just as Peter Jennings on "Days of Our Lives" or Jessie's husband on "All My Children." Her fears grew and grew until she became hysterical when her husband was gone unexpectedly or was late in returning from work or a business trip. She is now in psychiatric counseling to eliminate her unwarranted fears.

The promises of paradise here on earth, which are so prevalent in advertising, aren't found in the Bible. Instead Jesus assures us that we will have tribulation in this world. Then He adds, "but be of good cheer, I have overcome the world" (John 16:33).

It can be difficult for a woman to rise above the attitudes that surround her. Fortunately, we see our society's outlook gradually changing. We hope that more and more people will respect and revere older persons who have the wisdom and perspective of maturity and begin to recognize how many productive years lie beyond menopause. Then women will finally accept menopause for what it is: a developmental phase, which is part of the God-created seasons of our lives.

Chapter Twelve

DO I REALLY NEED A HYSTERECTOMY?

Hysterectomy! What an emotion-charged word for most women, whether they see it as a dreaded event, a frightening prospect, or a welcome relief.

Some of Orene's patients do all they can to avoid it. They forget appointments, ignore symptoms, ask for anything other than surgery. There's genuine panic in their eyes when Orene discusses the need for hysterectomy. Usually, some deep, underlying fear needs to be discussed. Most often it is not realistic.

Other patients come into the office after a long interval between visits and very little discussion about symptoms. They simply announce, "I'm tired of all this! I want a hysterectomy. Sign me up. This week, if you can." They've made up their minds before consulting Orene, who often responds gently, "Now wait a minute. I'm the one who needs to adjust to this!"

Still other women make an educated, well thought-out decision. These women come in for numerous appointments, try medication, and perhaps a D & C to correct their problems. When they've adjusted to the fact that a hysterectomy is the only way to achieve relief, "I'm ready," they say.

How will you know if you're ready for a hysterectomy? In years past, surgeons were often quick—perhaps too quick—to suggest a hysterectomy as the ultimate cure. After all, it was easier than working with a patient, month after month.

That's no longer true today, partly because women are more knowledgeable and more active in decision-making.

Insurance companies have also influenced the new attitude toward hysterectomies, since they now require preadmission certification, in which they review the reasons for surgery and approve the admission to the hospital. These companies often insist on a second opinion to make sure the surgery is indicated. (Medicare is also beginning to require preadmission certification before certain types of surgery.)

WHAT TO ASK YOUR DOCTOR ABOUT HYSTERECTOMY

It's your body, so you have every right to know why your physician feels surgery is necessary and what to expect.

Orene has prepared a video cassette, which explains the entire surgical procedure and includes slides from the operating room to help answer her patients' questions. She also gives them an opportunity to ask specific questions about what may be bothering or confusing them. In this chapter we will answer some questions you might ask your doctor and suggest a few others for you to ask, which will vary from physician to physician.

1. Why is a hysterectomy necessary?

If your doctor recommends this surgery, you may have any one of several benign conditions: fibroids, endometriosis, pelvic relaxations, or you may have a pre-cancer or even a cancer. Let's begin with the *growths that are benign.*

Fibroids are benign tumors of the muscle layer of the uterine wall. If you are having heavy menstrual periods (with clots or flooding) and/or bleeding between periods, you may have fibroids (see illustration 1). Another symptom is enlargement of the uterus which becomes irregular in shape. When a fibroid does not respond to medical management or to a D & C, surgery is indicated.

The only surgical alternative to a hysterectomy is a *my-*

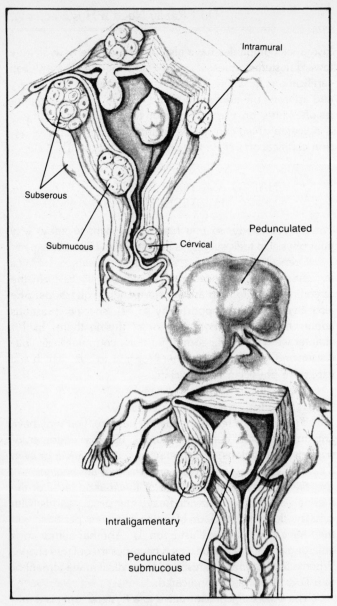

FIBROID TUMORS
Illustration 1

Benign uterine tumors, commonly called "fibroids," may be found in one fifth of women over 30 years of age.

omectomy, which is the removal of just the tumors and is quite complicated since the doctor will have to make an abdominal incision to take out the tumors, which are usually multiple in number. It should only be performed on a woman who wants to become pregnant afterwards, since this procedure entails a large amount of bleeding. Although this surgery will decrease the size of the uterus and allow the doctor to analyze the tissue, it may not alleviate the patient's pain and abnormal menstrual periods.

With *endometriosis,* the glandular tissue which lines the uterus is found outside the uterus, usually along the surface of the pelvic organs and ligaments. If you are experiencing pain and bleeding, you might also have endometriosis. Your doctor may suspect this condition after a pelvic exam and confirm the diagnosis by suggesting a laparoscopy, a minor surgical procedure in which a tube (the laparoscope) is inserted through a small incision in the navel and pushed into the abdominal cavity. In endometriosis, tiny implants of glandular tissue may appear on the ovaries, uterus, and connecting ligaments (see illustration 2). Your doctor will look at the surface of the pelvic organs to see these implants or any unsuspected chronic infection by viewing through a laproscope.

Adenomyosis (internal endometriosis) occurs when the glandular tissue is found in the muscle wall of the uterus, rather than outside the uterus. Remember, these glands should only be found lining the inner cavity of the uterus. This condition is painful and causes heavy periods. Adenomyosis cannot be definitely diagnosed until a hysterectomy is performed so the muscle layer can be studied microscopically; however, a doctor may suspect the presence of this condition if the uterus becomes slightly enlarged and soft.

Pelvic inflammatory disease is an infection of the fallopian tubes or ovaries. A gonorrhea infection or a more recently discovered venereal disease, chlamydia, sometimes leads to pelvic inflammatory disease. Chlamydia is a preva-

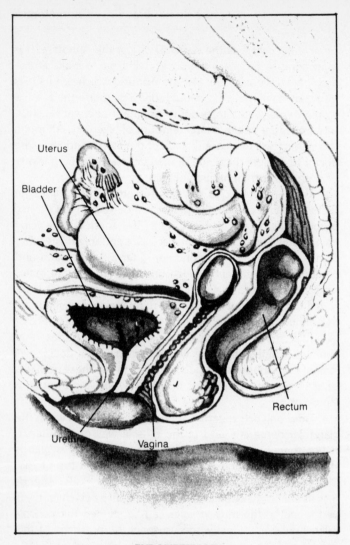

ENDOMETRIOSIS
Illustration 2

The tissue lining the uterine cavity is called the endometrium. When endometrial tissue occurs outside the uterine cavity, the disorder is called endometriosis.

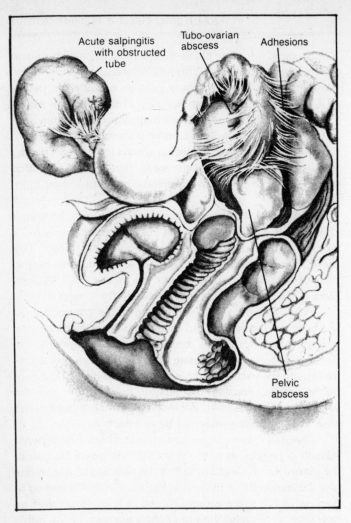

Acute salpingitis with obstructed tube

Tubo-ovarian abscess

Adhesions

Pelvic abscess

PELVIC INFLAMMATORY DISEASE
Illustration 3

Pelvic inflammatory disease (PID) results from infection of the pelvic structures by bacteria. Approximately three fourths of PID results from gonorrhea. Other causes are chlamydia, streptococcus, staphylococcus, or even bacteria normally found in the bowels.

lent bacterial infection of the fallopian tubes, which causes infertility and can lead to chronic, recurrent pelvic infection (see illustration 3). Very rarely does an intrauterine device (IUD) contribute to such an infection in the fallopian tubes.

Pelvic inflammatory disease may respond to antibiotics, but it often recurs, causing chronic discomfort. If this infection goes untreated and an abcess should form, it can be life-threatening. Most physicians agree that if this condition occurs over and over, a hysterectomy is the only way to insure a cure.

A doctor will also recommend surgery when the pain is chronic and debilitating. "I can't take this pain anymore," a woman sometimes declares. "I want a hysterectomy." This person needs to realize that the disease may not be curable without removal of the ovaries and the tubes as well. A complete "pelvic clean-out" is usually needed.

Pelvic Relaxation is a weakening of the connective tissue between the vagina and other organs. Sometimes hysterectomy is performed in conjunction with an operation to correct *cystocele,* a weakening of the bladder so that it protrudes into the vagina, and *rectocele,* weakening in the connective tissue, causing the rectum to protrude into the vagina (see illustration 4). If the uterus is not removed at this time, the procedures may not be as effective.

Uterine prolapse is the extreme condition where pelvic relaxation progresses to the point that the cervix (mouth of the uterus) protrudes to or out of the opening of the vagina (see illustration 5). A hysterectomy, along with tightening of the connective tissue around the vagina, or sometimes an operation to suspend the top of the vagina up in the pelvis will generally correct the problem.

Pelvic mass is an enlargement of a pelvic organ. Your doctor may find an enlargement of the ovary or uterus during a routine pelvic examination or from an ultrasound of the pelvis. Sometimes it is difficult to discern between a fibroid, which is part of the uterus, and an ovarian cyst, since the

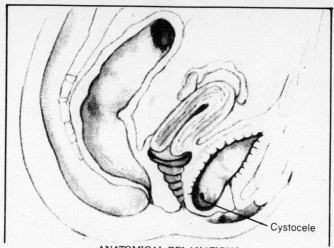

Cystocele

ANATOMICAL RELAXATIONS
Illustration 4

Cystocele, the protrusion of the urinary bladder into the vaginal wall, is often present because of the close proximity of the bladder to the vagina. Rectocele, the hernial protrusion of part of the rectum into the vagina, frequently accompanies prolapse because of laxity of pelvic floor structures.

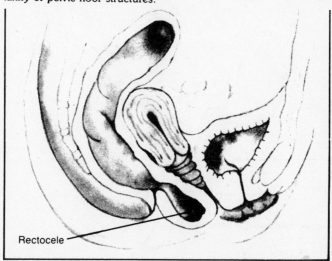

Rectocele

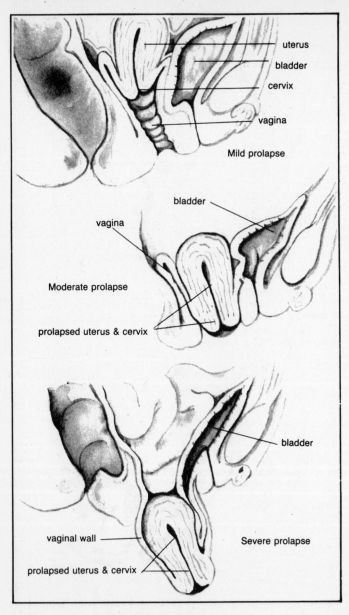

uterus

bladder

cervix

vagina

Mild prolapse

bladder

vagina

Moderate prolapse

prolapsed uterus & cervix

bladder

vaginal wall

Severe prolapse

prolapsed uterus & cervix

PROLAPSE OF THE UTERUS
Illustration 5

Prolapse of the uterus is any descent of the uterus below its normal position in the pelvis.

ovary can be located very close to the uterus.

In the postmenopausal woman, any enlargement is reason for an exploratory laparotomy to look at the surface of the pelvic organs. Usually the uterus is removed together with the ovaries. If a premenopausal woman has a solid pelvic mass or a large cystic mass that proves to be malignant, preparation should be made prior to surgery for hysterectomy, since it most often increases the chance of cure.

All of the problems we have considered so far are not cancerous. Now let's look at *precancerous growths and cancers.* We have already mentioned the stages that are thought to lead to cancer.

The first is *hyperplasia,* a change in the uterine lining, which is detectable by an endometrial biopsy, a microscopic examination of tissue removed from the lining. Hyperplasia is a benign change but is thought to lead to cancer if it progresses. If it does not disappear after the use of progesterone for six months or so, you should consider a hysterectomy.

Another type of precancer is *dysplasia of the cervix,* which is first suspected when a Pap smear is abnormal. The doctor can then visualize these cells under a microscope (called a "colposcope") and biopsy the lesion. Sometimes he or she will recommend a hysterectomy if a dysplasia is found.

However, the current trend is to try to preserve the uterus. One technique is cryosurgery (freezing the tissue), which is an office procedure. A newer technique is laser surgery, an outpatient procedure that evaporates the cells. Both have a high cure rate: ninety to ninety-six percent for laser surgery, and somewhat lower for cryosurgery. Laser surgery is more effective since viruses (especially the papilloma virus) are often associated with precancers, and the laser kills these viruses with more accuracy than other techniques.

In some cases, cone biopsy (taking a plug of tissue from the cervix) is performed in the hospital. This minor procedure may serve as therapy for the lesion, but it is mainly done as a diagnostic procedure. The risks include hemorrhage and infection, as well as the inability to maintain a pregnancy because of an incompetent cervix, a rare but serious complication.

If these treatments fail or the cervical lesion recurs, a hysterectomy may be the best alternative.

Only the most conservative doctors would treat *atypical adenomatous hyperplasia* medically with hormones, since it is a very definite precancer of the uterus. Most patients, except those who are in poor health and might die from the operative procedure, should have a hysterectomy.

Cancer of the uterus is, of course, a definite indication for hysterectomy, sometimes in conjunction with radiation therapy.

As we have discussed these reasons for a hysterectomy, we have also answered two other questions you may wish to ask a doctor: "What are the alternatives to a hysterectomy?" and "What will happen if I don't have surgery?"

2. Tell me, just what is a hysterectomy?

Most women realize that a hysterectomy means removing the uterus. However, a woman may have an option as to how much of the uterus is removed and what other organs are also taken (see illustration 6).

In a *subtotal hysterectomy* the uterus is removed leaving the cervix. Although subtotal hysterectomies were performed thirty years ago, the operation is rarely done today, because the cervix is a potential site for cancer and it is nonfunctional after a hysterectomy. Removing the cervix does not generally increase the complication of the surgery.

A *total hysterectomy*, the removal of both the uterus and the cervix, is a common form of hysterectomy that does not disturb hormonal function.

Hysterectomy with unilateral or bilateral salpingo-oophorectomy, the removal of one or both ovaries as well as the uterus and cervix, is often called a complete hysterec-

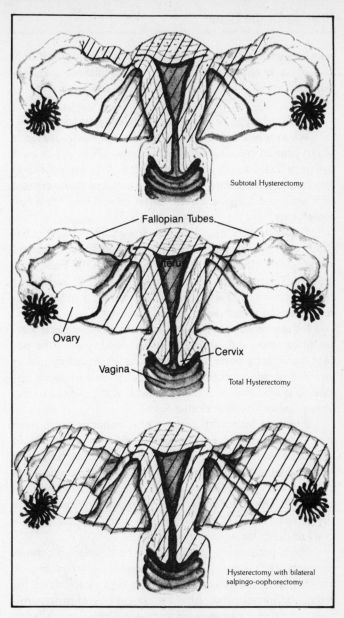

Subtotal Hysterectomy

Fallopian Tubes

Uterus

Ovary

Cervix

Vagina

Total Hysterectomy

Hysterectomy with bilateral
salpingo-oophorectomy

TYPES OF HYSTERECTOMY
(Shaded areas indicate the areas that are removed)
Illustration 6

tomy, which is not really a medical term. Obviously if only one ovary is removed the surgery is a unilateral salpingo-oophorectomy; if two are removed it is bilateral.

3. Which type of hysterectomy is the best for me?

When a hysterectomy is indicated, the next question is often: Should the ovaries also be removed? If you're over age forty-five, doctors often feel it's better to remove the ovaries than to leave them. The risk of ovarian cancer increases with age, and the ovaries will be functional for only a few more years.

Some doctors question this procedure, however, because even though the ovaries stop producing estrogen and progesterone, they still produce androgens (a male hormone) for many years. As we saw in chapter 2, androgens can be converted to estrogen in fatty tissue, a process that continues long after menopause.

If the ovaries are diseased and will possibly cause persistent symptoms, they should be removed, even if the patient is only forty years old or less. This is particularly true in the case of adhesion formation in pelvic inflammatory disease. It is also true with many tumors of the ovaries or the uterus, as well as in endometriosis.

If you are facing the decision of whether or not to have your ovaries as well as your uterus removed, you should know that ovarian cancer is one of the most lethal tumors. It is very silent as it develops, and greater than sixty percent of these cancers have spread outside the ovaries before they are found. The annual death rate from ovarian cancer in the United States is 10,000, and the risk is one percent (or one in a hundred) for women over forty.

Many patients are like Jackie, who developed ovarian problems twelve years after her vaginal hysterectomy. A sixty-two-year-old doctor's wife, she was hospitalized for vague abdominal pains. After evaluation by a gastroenterologist, who found no cause for the pains, Orene was called in and discovered a 6-centimeter, right ovarian cyst. Any cyst this large must be removed, since it can be cancerous. Fortunately this one was benign, but it's a typical illustration of what can happen when the ovaries are left in a middle-aged patient.

4. How will the operation be performed?

The uterus can be removed by two methods: a vaginal hysterectomy where the uterus is removed through the vagina without any incision and an abdominal hysterectomy where the uterus is removed through a surgical incision in the abdomen.

Today the *vaginal hysterectomy* is performed less often than the abdominal hysterectomy. It should not be considered if the uterus is enlarged and could not easily be brought out through the vagina, or if the physician is not certain whether or not the patient has adhesions, endometriosis, or a chronic infection. In these cases, the uterus may be very difficult to separate from vital organs, like the bowel and bladder, if a vaginal route is used.

The greatest problem with a vaginal hysterectomy is that it's "blind." There's a greater risk of blood loss, since the surgeon sometimes can't see to tie the adjacent structures as easily.

However, vaginal hysterectomy may be a good alternative if the uterus is normal in size and the patient has good relaxation of the pelvic organs, so they can easily be moved down. In addition, the surgeon must feel confident that there are no problems that might cause other organs to stick to the uterus as it's removed.

Often a vaginal hysterectomy is performed for a prolapse or "dropping down" of the pelvic organs and in conjunction with *colporraphy* (repair of vaginal tissues). This additional procedure is necessary when the pelvic organs relax and the bladder or rectum protrudes into the vagina, sometimes causing urinary leakage.

After the hysterectomy is performed, an incision is made through the vaginal tissues to expose the tough connective tissue. Then this tissue is brought tightly across the entire length of the vagina to support the bladder and rectum, so they no longer protrude into the vagina (see illustration 7). If the opening of the vagina is gaping or too relaxed, the surgeon will modify the size of the opening.

Some women prefer a vaginal hysterectomy because they want to avoid an abdominal scar. Orene often sees two other benefits of this surgery: her patients are better able to walk without pain immediately after surgery and they progress a bit quicker during the month after surgery, unless a complication occurs, such as infection of the operative site or excessive bleeding.

In an *abdominal hysterectomy,* the uterus is removed through an incision in the abdomen rather than through the vagina. The incision can be made transversely at the hairline, which makes the scar less visible, or it can be made vertically.

5. What are the possible complications of this surgery?

It's natural to assume that your surgery will be completely routine and that there will be no complications. The vast majority of surgeries do go smoothly. However, Orene likes to alert her patients to any possible complications beforehand, so that they will accept these complications better if they do happen. No woman likes negative surprises when she's already physically and emotionally depleted.

Medical problems of any major surgery can include respiratory complications of anesthesia, difficulties with the heart (such as a heart attack or arrhythmia), stroke, pulmonary embolus from phlebitis (or a blood clot in the leg), and even death. Certainly, these problems are more likely in the person who already has medical problems (such as heart disease or atherosclerosis) or has had a prior complication of this kind. In the healthy middle-aged person, the risks are very small.

Surgical complications include the possibility of hemorrhage and the necessity of transfusion. There is also some potential for infection after hysterectomy, since the surgeon enters the vagina, which contains bacteria, in order to remove the cervix. The operative site is, therefore, no longer sterile. Whereas the risk of infection was at one time thirty percent or so, physicians now often prescribe prophylactic antibiotics just before and for one day after surgery, which has reduced this figure by more than half.

A less common, but more serious complication, is the risk of perforating a vital organ such as the bowel or bladder during the surgery. This very unusual complication might occur if the patient has adhesions or if the uterus is distorted.

It may sound frightening to hear that a patient can die in surgery. But the risk of death from hysterectomy is only two-tenths of one percent (two per one thousand women), which includes the statistics of both healthy patients and very ill patients, some with far advanced cancers or other serious medical problems. In a healthy woman, the death rate is very close to zero.

The occurrence of any complications is also very small. We have come so far since the days of the first fifteen hysterectomies in the mid 1800s when only three women survived. Today hysterectomy is rarely life-threatening and can be life-saving.

6. How much time will I need to recuperate?

The rule of thumb is that any major surgery requires six weeks of recuperation before returning to full-time work. This time can vary, depending on the individual's ability to snap back, the kind of work, and whether or not there are any complications.

Remember you must heal both physically and emotionally. After surgery, you will feel how physically weak you are, but you may not sense the difference in your emotional strength. For instance, it may be very difficult to make decisions and accept responsibility. Most patients assume that the reason they cannot drive a car for three weeks is physical, but it is also because you are not adept at making split-second decisions.

If the surgery is elective, plan to have other help with the cooking, cleaning, and laundry. Some things can be done ahead, but don't wear yourself out in an effort to cover the work of your entire recuperation period just before surgery. At times, it's helpful to have a relative or someone with whom you feel very comfortable stay with you for the week after you return from the hospital, especially if you have younger children with multiple needs.

The process of recuperation can be hastened if you'll make the effort to walk, first at home and, after a week, outside. Increase the distance gradually, depending on your stamina, and be sure to do your initial outside walking with someone else. It will be an effort to stand straight at first, but make it your goal, even while you're still in the hospital. Remember, it's not safe to lift anything heavier than ten pounds for up to six weeks after your surgery.

You may have minor problems with gas and bowel movements for the first week or two after hysterectomy. Walking, and sometimes taking laxatives or stool softeners, will help these difficulties. You may also feel some mild burning with urination, some pain in the lower abdomen when emptying a full bladder, and some hesitancy in initiating urination. These problems should clear without any particular medication, unless an accompanying infection has begun.

You may also notice a sense of fullness and loss of sensation in the vaginal area during the recuperation period. Orene's aerobic exercise instructor emphasizes the use of Kegel exercises (see chapter 4) in restoring the normal sensation and muscle control of the vaginal tissues. In fact, she feels that this exercise is important in maintaining healthy vaginal musculature in any woman and recommends that "Kegels" be done forever.

7. Will I need estrogen?

The answer is no, if the ovaries, or even one ovary, are left intact. If you also have your ovaries removed, with few exceptions, estrogen therapy is a must if you have not yet been through menopause. Some doctors prescribe progesterone as well; some do not.

Surgeons once thought it better for a woman to get through the adjustments and symptoms of surgical menopause without estrogens. That's generally no longer true. There really is no point in withholding estrogen. Forty-eight hours after a hysterectomy the estrogen in the system will have metabolized, and a woman will be uncomfortable. She develops a fairly rapid rise in her FSH and experiences immediate hot flushes and perhaps headaches. Her symptoms are exaggerated, compared with the woman experiencing a natural menopause, because she is suddenly and prematurely, deprived. Within a few years, as we have seen, she may develop vaginal changes and she is at very high risk for osteoporosis.

The estrogen dosage for a woman after surgical menopause may be no different than the supplement for postmenopausal women, usually in the range of .625 milligrams to 1.25 milligrams per day of conjugated estrogen. As we mentioned in chapter 5, progesterone may also be given for ten days of the month.

Unless there are serious side effects, estrogen replacement therapy should continue until the mid-fifties. At that time, doctors usually begin to wean a patient from the drug to see if hot flushes return or if they are minimal. Since physicians do not know how long it takes to minimize osteoporosis after surgical menopause, there is not a well-defined time to stop hormone replacement.

8. What if you've had only your uterus removed?

If you have a hysterectomy prior to menopause, you lose your monitoring device, your uterus. Since you no longer menstruate, you don't see the change in your periods as you approach menopause or their ultimate cessation.

Yet you still have your ovaries, so you may still notice monthly or cyclic hormonal changes, such as tender breasts and premenstrual tension. You will also experience menopause just like your sister who did not have a hysterectomy, but perhaps slightly earlier. You may find yourself surprised by menopausal symptoms, or you may not even recognize them for what they are. An FSH test will tell you and your doctor if you are in menopause and help you decide what treatment might be desirable.

9. Will I feel any emotional side effects?

For some women, the emotional trauma of hysterectomy, particularly if the ovaries are removed, is far greater than the physical, especially for younger women.

"It's too soon," one patient repeated, again and again. There can be a tremendous sense of deprivation in the finality of "no babies," or even "no more babies." Sometimes these feelings are intensified by a sense of lost womanhood and even loss of identity as a woman. Fears of loss of sexuality and sexual response loom darkly. "I feel I'm being castrated," one patient confessed before her surgery. Depression can be intense.

Much of the emotional pain can be prevented, however, by adequate psychological preparation for the surgery. It's important, as we've noted, for a woman to express her concerns, ask questions, and receive answers from her doctor.

Often it helps to go through the thought process of dealing with the loss of reproductive function beforehand. Of course, one can't complete the grief process before a death occurs, but a woman can do a lot of the ground work, so that all the emotions don't strike at once.

Most women adjust easily to surgical menopause, as long as they understand that it will not reduce their femininity or their sexuality. If the ovaries are removed, a woman will not age any more rapidly than if she still has her ovaries, if hormone supplements are taken.

Some women, like Gwen, have been programmed to expect emotional problems after a hysterectomy. In fact, Gwen's mother, who did not take estrogens after surgery and experienced emotional trauma, told her, "If you have a hysterectomy, make sure you don't have the ovaries removed."

Gwen had such pain from endometriosis, Orene could not guarantee that her ovaries could be left intact. Once Gwen understood that hormone replacement would have eliminated most of her mother's problems, she felt comfortable about the surgery. Her ovaries and uterus were removed, but she experienced a smooth transition and rapid recuperation with hormone therapy.

Nancy, a forty-one-year-old secretary, had a similar fear of emotional changes, since her husband's mother committed suicide a few years after a hysterectomy. Apparently the mother-in-law had some prior episodes of depression, but the family blamed the surgery for her death. What a heavy burden to pass down to the next generation!

Nancy suffered from very heavy menstrual periods associated with multiple but small fibroids. At this point, Nancy has only had a D & C, but Orene is not sure that she will achieve significant improvement in her bleeding pattern, since medical therapy, such as hormones, will not help her problem.

The most important part of her treatment is to begin to deal with her fear of hysterectomy. Orene has suggested that she and her husband read a booklet on hysterectomy, printed by the American College of Obstetricians and Gynecologists, and talk to women who have had hysterectomies.

Then Orene has asked to talk to them together to help them gain confidence that if Nancy has the surgery she will not have severe emotional problems.

10. Would a second opinion be a good idea?

Your insurance company may require a second opinion for preadmission certification. Or your own physician may suggest it in order to clarify the need for the surgery to you and your family, especially if you are uncertain about the decision.

You may also feel the desire to have a second opinion, just for reassurance. The protocol is to discuss it with your primary physician, rather than to sneak out behind her or his back. You might say, "Doctor, this is such a big decision for me and my family that I would like to have a second opinion before I schedule my surgery with you. Could you make any suggestions, and do you need to send that doctor any communication or records?"

11. How much will this cost?

Be sure to ask what the surgeon's bill will be and that of any assisting physician. Remember, too, there will be a fee for the anesthesiologist and possibly for a cardiologist, if an electrocardiogram is performed.

Many insurance agencies pay eighty percent of a usual customary fee which *they* set. Thus, it is wise to call them first to find how much you may actually be expected to pay. The total bill may be as much as five to six thousand dollars, so it's important to know approximately what percentage you will have to pay.

12. I am particularly fearful of —, and I want to know if this is likely to be a problem.

Don't be afraid to express your anxieties, whatever they may be. The most common ones seem to be fear of obesity, growth of excess facial hair, lack of libido, and "going off the deep end." *None* of these is an inevitable outcome of a hysterectomy.

Many times your husband may want to be involved in the surgical consultation. Certainly it's all right to bring him, but make sure you schedule his visit. It is particularly important to involve husbands if you're having difficulty making some of the decisions, if your husband has different ideas from yours, if he has been misinformed, or if he has questions and fears about the surgery.

One husband, for instance, had heard from the "guys at work" that hysterectomy could alter his wife's sexual response and that she wouldn't have the same feelings for him. This myth is not uncommon, and the most important factor is to deal with it before surgery. Orene makes a point of sitting down with the couple, to reassure them and educate them about the very few ways that hysterectomy might change their relationship. To fail to settle these issues before surgery can allow room for false blame and breakdown of relationships, which takes much more work to restore once it's occurred. Although there may be some correlation between disfiguring cancer cases and disruption of marriage, we know of no study that suggests an increase in divorce after hysterectomy.

13. Will my sexual response change after a hysterectomy?

We've already answered this question, except for the one possible exception, which is atrophic vaginitis, a condition we discussed in chapters 3, 4, 5, and 6.

Meryl was a lovely blonde in her late forties who had a hysterectomy with the removal of her ovaries several years before Orene saw her. During the past six months, she had felt so much pain with intercourse that she and her husband had stopped trying for two months. She said her husband was very understanding, but she wondered what was wrong.

Orene found that Meryl had a great deal of thinning and dryness of vaginal tissues, a delayed side effect of her surgery. After six weeks of oral estrogen, she came back to the office to report that her symptoms were gone. "Deep down, I felt there was some dark, psycho-sexual meaning to my problem," she admitted. "I never dreamed I'd find such a simple and satisfactory answer."

14. What should I do to prepare for surgery?

A. Call your insurance company. Ask if you are covered for this surgery, if any preadmission review or second opinion is required, and how much the company will pay.

B. Get plenty of rest before the operation. Resist the temptation to do two months' worth of work during the few days preceding your admission to the hospital.

C. Exercise. If surgery is elective, you may have time to get yourself into better condition through exercise. However, this can't be approached as a rush job. Orene's patients who have been exercising regularly and have not allowed themselves to become obese recover easily.

D. Talk to other women who have had this surgery, but choose carefully. Look for someone who will be reassuring. Who needs a tale of horror from someone who experienced major complications?

E. Check the possibility of autotransfusion. In some communities, you can give a unit of your own blood two-to-three weeks before surgery, which is saved for the date of your surgery if it should be needed. This precaution offers protection from the possibility of AIDS or hepatitis. This effort is not advisable, if you're already anemic or if you're likely to need a greater quantity of blood. It's also not realistic for you to stockpile more than one or two units, because it will not be replenished in your own body by the surgery date, and it only can be stored in the blood bank for thirty days.

15. How long will the procedure take?

The length of the operation varies, depending on the disease process and the technical difficulty of the surgery; however, it is generally one and one-half to two hours. Contrast this to the three to four hours that is not uncommon for cancer surgery and for surgery for prolapse of the uterus.

16. What kind of anesthesia will be used?

Usually a general anesthesia is given for a hysterectomy.

17. How long will I be hospitalized?

Patients must remain in the hospital until they are self-sufficient, can take solid foods, and are off all intramuscular medication. The hospitalization varies from five to seven days if there are no complications. If an infection or some other complication occurs, then the hospital stay may be several days longer.

If you are facing hysterectomy, you may be like the countless women who declare, "I know I need it, but I'm scared to death."

The best medicine for you is to make a list of the steps we have suggested and check them off as you complete them. When you have finished, in all likelihood, you will no longer be afraid of what lies ahead.

If, however, some small doubts and fears surface when you're alone, or in the darkness of night, remember how Jehoshaphat's army approached its battle, singing and praising God and believing in His mercy (2 Chron. 20).

You will probably join the many, many patients who feel so much better after surgery. Often they wonder why they hesitated and wish they'd scheduled it much sooner!

Chapter Thirteen

"THE BOTTOM LINE IS THE LORD"

"You know what made all the difference in my experience with menopause?" a handsome salt-and-pepper-haired woman asked. "I learned in the very beginning that the bottom line is the Lord. Sure, you see your doctor, and you hope for support and understanding from your family and friends. But they're all human. They can't always give you what you need. God's the one you can always count on."

For countless women, the bottom line at this time of life is the Lord. But what does that mean? How can He help us to cope with menopause? What does Scripture tell us about handling this time of life?

Can there really be "joy in all things?"

A Bible study on the Book of Philippians changed the focus of the woman we just mentioned. "I wasn't exactly comfortable, to say the least, with the hot flashes and emotional ups and downs," she admitted. "But suddenly I realized that the apostle Paul was never comfortable! Yet he could tell us to 'rejoice in all things.' I wondered if that was truly possible."

Then came one of those ghastly days we've all experienced. After a night of fitful sleep, she'd clashed with another woman at work. Reviewing the conversation as she left the office, she felt guilty over how unreasonable she'd been. She arrived home to start dinner and found that her teenager had consumed the left-over roast she had planned to serve. Well, then, she'd whip up a cheese soufflé. But when she checked it half an hour later, she found that it hadn't puffed at all.

"I can't believe this!" she muttered to herself as she opened the refrigerator to see what else she might prepare—and knocked the salad dressing out onto the tile floor. The bottle shattered. Near tears now, she began to pick up the glass, cut her hand, and dripped blood, oil, and vinegar on her camel colored wool skirt. Just then her son appeared, and asked, "Is dinner ready?"

"No!" she shouted. On the brink of exploding at him, she stormed down the hall, slammed the front door, and began stalking furiously down the street.

"I wasn't sure how far I was going, but I knew I had to get out of there," she recalled. "I was crying, telling myself it wasn't fair. 'Lord,' I said, 'did I deserve all that?' "

After a few blocks, she slowly began to remember her study of Philippians. Paul had said, "I know how to be abased, and I know how to abound....I can do all things through Christ who strengthens me" (Phil. 4:12, 13). "At last," she recalled, "I said, 'Lord, through your grace, I can do this. In fact, I *will* rejoice in this. Not for it. But in it.' " Then, a few moments later, she could honestly add, "I love You. I praise You. I trust You."

In another two blocks, she felt "an amazing serenity. I even knew I could face cleaning up the salad dressing and the glass."

When she returned home, she found that her son had picked up most of the glass. Then the thought occurred to her that she could serve the unpuffed soufflé over toast.

There is a depth of peace and joy that can surpass everyday frustration, as this woman discovered; but sometimes it takes getting off alone with God to find it again.

Basically, joy is a choice. We can learn to be joyful in all things, or as James suggested, to "count it all joy" when we meet various trials. Frequently, we see David making a choice. He begins many a Psalm with deep despair, "My

God, My God, why have You forsaken Me?" (Ps. 22:1). He had good cause, for King Saul, the Philistines, many people were out for his head.

After recounting his troubles, David is not afraid to plead with God for help, just as we can. "O My Strength, hasten to help Me....Save Me from the lion's mouth" (Ps. 22:19-21).

"You have answered Me," he asserts at the end of that verse.

David gives the secret of his ability to carry on in the midst of trouble in Psalm 130:

I wait for the LORD, my soul waits,
And in his word I do hope.
My soul waits for the LORD
More than those who watch for the morning...
O Israel, hope in the LORD. (vv. 5-7)

Two words are critical here: *wait* and *hope*. David was willing to wait for God to act in his life, just as a watchman waited for the dawn of morning light. How long does a watchman wait? All night, despite fatigue and the unrest of boredom. What else does he do? Little else, but sit and watch and wait, only walking around the plant or office building once an hour to check the premises.

David could wait in this way, he says, because God's Word gave him hope. Waiting with hope—this is David's secret of getting through tough times. It may be yours, too. What about reading the promises in the Bible as you wait for your emotions to settle? You could buy a book of these promises, such as *The Personal Promise Pocketbook*.

Bev found that the promise in Isaiah 46:4 really spoke to her during menopause. "I will be your God through all your lifetime, yes, even when your hair is white with age. I made you and I will care for you. I will carry you along and be your Savior" (TLB).

To keep this focus, author and lecturer Anne Ortlund once told how she lettered a large sign, which read Alleluia!, and placed it on the floor just where her feet touch each morning when she rolls out of bed. A neighbor who requires regular dialysis because of kidney disease, revealed that each day when she gets up, she pulls the drapes, looks out the window, and says two words, "Thanks, Lord."

About Your Attitude

In the last chapter, we discussed the attitudes of others and how they may affect us, and we concluded that as Christians we need not accept the attitudes of the world. What, then, should be our attitude?

The Book of Philippians addresses this in chapter 2, verse 5: "Let this mind (The New International Version reads "attitude") be in you which was also in Christ Jesus." The verse goes on to explain that Jesus' "mind" or "attitude" was that of a servant. For He was willing to humble Himself and be obedient, even unto death. Therefore God has highly exalted Him. So the way *up* for Jesus was *down* first.

Can we use this time of our lives to learn this lesson in humility—to "humble yourselves under the mighty hand of God, that He may exalt you in due time" (1 Pet. 5:6)?

We believe that we can if we remember whom we must serve first. We serve God first, just as Jesus did. If we try to serve people first, we will surely be disappointed, for we'll never completely please them. But we can please God by serving others.

One of the most unforgettable women we know taught a neighborhood Bible study in Southern California, which attracted many young women who had never opened a Bible before. When she became ill with cancer, she insisted upon continuing the study. Chemotherapy destroyed her glorious head of hair, her face grew thin and drawn. Finally, she was hospitalized, but she left the hospital for two hours each week to lead the Bible study. "I gain more than those I teach," she insisted when her doctors questioned this weekly departure, although her study group would argue with that. She taught the Bible study just a few days before she died.

Do you see what happens when we focus on pleasing God, not ourselves? We stop dwelling on our own problems. We become useful both to Him and to others—and to ourselves.

"Yes, but I'm so miserable!"

Strong's Concordance lists ninety biblical references to *suffering* (in the sense of hurting). Ninety! Plus seventeen uses of the word *anguish* and thirty-six of *pain.* Do those words make you wince? How often most of us pray, "Don't let it hurt, Lord!"

Unfortunately, many Christians seem to believe that they shouldn't suffer. "If my faith was great enough, I wouldn't feel like this," they say. Or, "Surely I'm not a good Christian or I wouldn't be having all these difficulties."

Where, we wonder, is that written? Not in the Bible. The truth is that Christians have no guarantee of freedom from inner conflict, physical pain, or other stressful events. That's life, in biblical times and today. The Bible clearly tells us again and again that we will suffer.

Let's stop ignoring the passages about suffering and remember that God gives us vast spiritual resources to draw upon. They will help us endure. They will help us overcome.

A neighbor of Bev's, Shannon, appeared to glow with health as she pursued a vigorous schedule of tennis and running. Then, suddenly, rheumatoid arthritis struck this beautiful, dark-haired woman. For many weeks, her days were limited to rest and therapy.

She later told Bev, "Christians are so afraid of suffering, but I know now that I can find the Lord in the midst of my pain, and that His grace is sufficient either to lift me above the pain or to give me peace in the midst of it. The Lord has given me a courage I never thought I could have, and indeed, I didn't have it until I needed it."

You face into the wind, not denying adversity but yielding and trusting and believing that whatever He allows is for your good, she says, even though she knows she probably faces a lifetime of pain from her affliction. Think how short-lived our discomfort at menopause really is, in comparison!

If we view menopause as a time of refining, knowing that we are growing in God's image, we can see some purpose in this change and its discomfort. It truly can be a change for the better. Our spiritual resources can help us cope with our discomforts, just as they did the women we interviewed.

Dealing with Fear

A woman named Gloria told us that as she approached menopause, she felt almost paralyzed by the memory of her mother's very difficult time and by the fears which her mother projected upon her. She was afraid of emotional upheaval and physical discomfort.

"Then, one day, I realized that I had a choice," she recalls. "I could see my body as an enemy and could focus on all the ways it might hurt me. Or I could release all that to God and focus on His love. You know what? It's impossible to think of two things at the same time!"

Gloria actually made the same decision as the psalmist when he wrote, "Whenever I am afraid, I will trust in You" (Ps. 56:3). And she also echoed the song of praise in Isaiah 12:2: "Behold, God is my salvation, I will trust and not be afraid. For...the LORD, is my strength and my song; He also has become my salvation."

What is it that you fear most about menopause? The emotional ups and downs? The physical symptoms? The fact that it indicates you're growing older?

If you center on that fear, it tends to magnify and the tension grows, intensifying whatever symptoms you might be feeling. But consider the perfect love, which was manifested in Jesus; doesn't the Bible tell us that perfect love will cast out our fear (1 John 4:18)?

Moreover, Paul states in Romans 8:14-15 that "For as many as are led by the Spirit of God, these are sons of God. For you did not receive the spirit of bondage again to fear, but you received the Spirit of adoption."

In other words, the old fear patterns of our lives before we knew the Lord are no longer valid today. We can rest in the perfect security of our Father's everlasting arms; even if we are born pessimists, we needn't expect the worst. And that's true even if we were raised by parents who programmed us to believe that the past was terrible, this moment is dreadful, and what comes next will be even worse.

We love the poster that proclaims: "Do you not know that what died on the cross was fear?" We pray that you will allow your fear to die as you meditate on the assurance that nothing can estrange you from the love of God. "For I am persuaded that neither death nor life, nor angels nor principalities nor powers, nor things present *nor things to come,* (italics ours) nor height nor depth, nor any other created thing, shall be able to separate us from the love of God which is in Christ Jesus our Lord" (Rom. 8:38-39).

Dealing with Feelings of Shame

Rodale's *Synonym Finder* equates shame with feeling debased, demeaned, unworthy. From time to time, these feelings may assault you as you go through this time of transition. Perhaps it will help you to remember that your body is His temple. It is not in any way defiled by these changes. In no way do they make you a lesser person.

"Behold," says the Lord in Isaiah 43:19, "I will do a new thing." And that is exactly what He does for us at this time of our lives. Can't we take joy in looking forward to this "new thing" with hope, remembering that we are still "fearfully and wonderfully made" by God's own design?

It is appropriate to ask ourselves if any shame we might

feel could be rooted in pride. Proverbs 11:2 states, "When pride comes, then comes shame," and sometimes we do tend to become overly obsessed with our youthfulness and beauty, to the point of narcissism. And that, strictly defined, means an extreme of self-love. Remember how the Greek god, Narcissus, fell in love with his own reflection?

Dealing with Feelings of Ugliness

It's important, of course, for us to take care of ourselves and our appearance. But it's sad when women become so depressed with what they see as the ravages of age that they seek extreme measures to turn back the clock. A few years ago Bev interviewed a surgeon for an article on plastic surgery. He proudly showed before-and-after pictures of an aging actress who had come to him for a face lift. The trouble was, Bev thought the "before" picture was the winner. The crinkles around the woman's eyes reflected years of smiles. The gentle countenance mirrored experience and fostered trust; the woman looked like a grandmother you could love. The "after" picture showed a woman whose skin was so tautly stretched, she looked insensitive and harsh, not young.

Of course, many of us are not altogether thrilled with what gravity is doing to our faces or our bodies. Even those of us who can say our measurements are the same may find them lower! But what, after all, is true beauty? The apostle Peter ascribed beauty to Sarah, who we suspect was still beautiful when she conceived Isaac at age ninety. Her beauty? The unfading beauty of "a gentle and quiet spirit." The beauty of the inner self, "which is very precious in the sight of God" (1 Pet. 3:4).

This beauty is what leads a son to tell his fifty-six-year-old mother, "You know, you're better looking now than you were ten years ago." This is the beauty that prompts Bev's father-in-law to say of his eighty-five-year-old wife, "I thought

Jessie was the prettiest girl in the world when I first saw her. And she still is!"

Dealing with Confusion

Certainly education helps dispel the confusion many women feel about menopause and the uncertainty over what will happen next. The more we understand the process we're undergoing, the less bewildered and unbalanced we're likely to feel. Still, there may be days of, "Stop this merry-go-round. I want to get off!"

How reassuring it is, then, to consider the very nature of God. You might try something Bev does when she is involved in something that's very repetitive, such as exercising or doing household tasks. Go through the alphabet, fitting an attribute of God to each letter and reminding yourself of His sovereignty. Just think, for instance, how long your list can be when you get to the letter "O". Consider His *omnipotence* (His unlimited, infinite power); His *omnipresence* (His unbounded, universal presence everywhere); His *omniscience* (His knowledge of all things). Ponder His *order* (the marvelous organization He manifests in all that He creates, from the world and its creatures to His very Word). As we dwell on Him, our confusion vanishes.

A friend of Bev's recently exclaimed, "When I step back and look at who He is and what He has done, I know what's happening to me now is not an accident, but part of His perfect plan. He created me female. He's given a natural rhythm to the seasons of life. There truly is 'a time to sow and a time to reap.' If we'll just go with them, how much happier we'll be!"

Dealing with Depression

"I'm so depressed," a woman admitted to her Bible study group recently, "I can't even pray."

"Oh, Mary," a member of the group responded immediately, "I'm so grateful you told us. Because, you see, it's OK.

We'll pray *for* you." And they did.

If you're feeling in the pits, don't keep it to yourself and try to be a silent, stoic Mrs. Job. Of course, we don't recommend the ashes and sackcloth approach, or moaning "Woe is me!" to everyone you meet. But do admit your despair to friends who care about you. Ask them to pray for you. We've seen miraculous results from such supplications, and the side effects, unlike those of many medications, are all positive.

Another approach to handling depression is to see if you can find the roots of the mental process which led you there. Peggy expressed her low times this way: "I look at the way I tend to lose my temper and/or my patience, and I immediately say to myself, 'Look at you! What a sterling example you are of the patient, kind Christian!' And then I become *really* depressed."

The turning point for Peggy was an Easter Bible study, which focused upon the historical record of the Resurrection. "If you feel you're not living the Christian life well, you must run to the objective events and put your faith *there*, not in yourself and your performance," the teacher urged.

Peggy confessed her failings to the Lord, admitted to Him and herself that her performance would never be "worthy," and centered herself upon the risen Christ. In Him is her power for living, her antidote to self-focused, self-defeating depression.

Another woman realized that her depression stemmed from a sense that life was essentially over for her. "I just didn't see much future," she explained. "The kids are gone, and my husband's a workaholic who's never going to retire. I learned later that the younger women in my Bible study called me 'the woman with the sad countenance.' "

It was not until she began a study of Moses that she realized she had a choice. The Lord charged Moses: "I call heaven and earth as witnesses today against you, that I have set before you life and death, blessing and cursing; therefore *choose* life, that both you and your descendants may live; that you may love the LORD your God, that you may obey His voice, and that you may cling to Him, for He is your life" (Deut. 30:19-20, italics ours).

She remembers, "I was amazed to see that I, too, could choose. But I had to make that choice, not just once and for all, but moment by moment, yielding to Him." Today, the Lord *is* her life. And what a difference He makes!

Psalm 77 might well be the cry of a menopausal woman:

> I cry to the Lord; I call and call to him. Oh, that he would listen. I am in deep trouble and I need his help so badly. All night long I pray, lifting my hands to heaven, pleading. . . .
>
> I keep thinking of the good old days of the past, long since ended. Then my nights were filled with joyous songs. I search my soul and meditate upon the difference now. (vv. 1-6, TLB)

The psalmist goes on to wonder, "Has the Lord rejected me forever? Will he never again be favorable? Has he slammed the door in anger on his love?"

Finally he makes the decision to count his blessings: "I recall the many miracles he did for me so long ago. Those wonderful deeds are constantly in my thoughts. . . . O God, your ways are holy. You are the God of miracles and wonders!" (vv. 11-14). At last, he is able to worship a God who is holy, great, and performs miracles to redeem his people.

Have you made a list of blessings lately? A list of the deeds of the Lord for you and your family? Look back over the last week. Can you see God's hand in the events? Maybe an answered prayer for a hurting daughter or a business opportunity your husband didn't expect?

Now review the last month, the last year. Finally, take a look at your entire life. Has God helped you through some difficult times? With your husband? Your kids? A readjustment you made, like going back to work?

Yes, you say, God has helped me in the past. If that's

so, can't you trust Him now? And in the future? Remember David's words: *wait* and *hope.*

Sometimes you can't pinpoint a specific cause for your depression. You simply *are depressed.* Then it may be difficult to be patient with those who think they can "jolly you out of it" (nothing seems funny at this point), or those who try to divert you with a movie or an ice cream soda (that's not what you want or need, at all).

Myra expressed it this way: "It was as though a switch had been pulled. For no apparent reason, suddenly, I was so low. I began to think that I must be mentally ill. And then I sank into the depths of self-pity."

One help to her at this time was a book on the various names of God. One of the names is *Jehovah Rapha,* "the Lord that heals."

"That name captivated my mind. And although these depressions continued to strike from time to time, it let me know that the God who made me could also restore me."

Whether you find yourself just feeling blue or hitting rock bottom, perhaps some of David's "pits to praises" psalms might be helpful at this time. Try Psalms 6, 13, and 22 for starters. God truly inhabits our praises, and depression does flee when we praise Him.

Dealing with Anger

Doris claims that Anglo Saxons are historically either farmers or fighters, that her husband is a farmer, she, a fighter. It's easy for her to feel rebellious and combative, she says, and menopause simply intensified her natural bent.

Many of us find our tempers and temperaments magnified at this time. Unfortunately, we may turn our resentment in the wrong direction, making those we love most the victims of the anger which simmers inside us.

If you find yourself lashing out at others, try meditating on Ephesians 4:20-32. Here Paul urges the Ephesians, "If you have really heard his [Christ's] voice and learned from

him the truths concerning himself, then throw off your old
evil nature....

"Now your attitudes and thoughts must all be constantly
changing for the better" (TLB). Notice that matter of attitude
again as he adds, "Stop being mean, bad-tempered and angry." And we would add, do it now, before it escalates!

But what if, despite all your prayers and good inten-
tions, you still blow? It's important then to remember that
God didn't choose us because we are holy, but that we might
be holy. We're still in process, and holiness is the beauty
which is gradually produced by His workmanship in us. Remember, too, the assurance of Psalm 130:3: "If You, LORD,
should mark iniquities, O LORD, who could stand? But there
is forgiveness...."

Dealing with Loneliness

Sometimes, during these middle years, the sense of
aloneness can be overwhelming. You *know* that no one else
feels the way you do. No one really understands what you're
going through. And most of all, you wonder why others
can't demonstrate just a little more patience and understanding toward you at this difficult time. We women seem to
have a special gift for laying expectations on others. *Surely,*
we think, they will respond to us with concern and caring.
Surely they'll step in and volunteer to help with difficult
tasks. And when they don't, we feel forsaken and lonely. We
set ourselves up for such disappointment, either by being totally unrealistic in what we expect or by failing to express our
needs. We structure a no-win situation.

It was only after many years of disappointment and
loneliness over unfulfilled expectations that Betty found the
verse, "My soul, wait silently for God alone, For my expectation is from Him. He only is my rock... my defense; I shall
not be moved" (Ps. 62:5-6). Indeed, God is the only safe,
sure person in whom we can place our expectations. He's
told us that He will never leave us or forsake us. He's prom-

ised us that He will be with us always, to the end of the world.

Dealing with Sleeplessness

Sometimes, despite prayer, warm milk, and a comfortable bed, sleep just doesn't come. Or we may waken much too early. Joyce told us that for months she struggled with these wakeful times until it occurred to her that this was "found" time alone with the Lord. And as she began exploring Scripture, she discovered what she terms "Psalms for Insomniacs." They reminded her that she should be glad if, "My eyes are awake through the night watches, That I may meditate on Your Word" (Ps. 119:148). And she began using this time to meditate on God's promises to her. At night, when she really sought God's help, the words of the Psalms came to life in a very personal way.

She learned from Psalms, too, to count her blessings instead of sheep. And in Psalm 16:7-9, she read, "I will bless the LORD who has given me counsel; My heart also instructs me in the night seasons....Because He is at my right hand I shall not be moved. Therefore my heart is glad, and my glory rejoices; My flesh also will rest in hope."

As you can see, the recurring theme in dealing with these negative emotions and situations is to choose to focus on the Lord. He will, as John Greenleaf Whittier wrote, "reclothe us in our rightful mind." He will help you and teach you through this time.

So like the apostle Paul, let's strive to be content in whatever state, and at whatever age we may be, not looking back on what is gone, but rejoicing in what we have, and looking forward to what will be. For if we believe in a God who loves us unconditionally and who is committed to what is best for us, our future is truly unlimited.

Chapter Fourteen

CELEBRATING YOUR FREEDOM

Whether your menopause is as placid as a reflecting pool or as turbulent as the seas off the tip of Cape Horn, you'll probably feel an enormous sense of relief and release when it's over.

It's true, of course, that you're no longer *reproductive*, but you're now wonderfully free to be *productive*, and you'll very likely experience a replenished vigor. Said one fifty-five-year-old, "I feel like I can overpower lions, and I have the experience to do it!" There's life—lots of it—after menopause. In fact, with today's longer life expectancy, you may have as much as half of your life still ahead of you.

One woman calculated her lifespan from a medical table and told her children, "I hate to break this to you, but according to this, I'll live to be a hundred and five." They moaned and groaned, of course, and one son said, "You mean I could still have you around when I'm an eighty-year-old kid?"

Even though we may not all have fifty years ahead of us, certainly most of us in menopause have thirty or more years to look forward to.

How will we use that time, that renewed energy and freedom? What a marvelous, infinite variety of options we have, more than ever before in history.

Free to Laugh and Play

Evidence on the healing, life-prolonging aspects of laughter and play is beginning to accumulate in the scientific community. But Solomon knew almost three thousand years ago that "A merry heart does good, like medicine, but a broken spirit dries the bones" (Prov. 17:22). He also perceived that "he who is of a merry heart has a continual feast" (Prov. 15:15).

Menopause may have been a serious business to you, but now's the time to cultivate your sense of humor, which may have fallen into disrepair in recent months and years. Where is it written that Christians must always be so somber? You might start by bringing a smile to those who need it most: women who are still in the grips of menopause. Send them a clever greeting card. Take them to a funny movie. Find out what's truly *fun* for them. (Mark Twain described fun as what you do when you don't have to do it.) Whether it's tennis or a drive to a special discount outlet, do it with them. Help them, too, to laugh at themselves and their symptoms.

One woman did just this by sending a bit of doggeral to a friend:

> A salesman called to sell a sauna
> And I replied, "I'm not a-gonna.
> Instead of shelling out the cash
> I'll sweat it out with a good hot flash!"

Another woman likes to lighten the day for family members. She knew just what to do after her husband came home with pavement burns all along his arm from a skidding wipe-out on his bike. The next day while he was at work, she equipped his sophisticated ten-speed racing bicycle with children's training wheels.

Still another keeps her sense of humor honed by practicing snappy comebacks to jokes about her age. For instance, when a doctor asked her, "What can you expect of that knee at your age?" she replied, "The other one's the same age and it's OK." And when an insurance agent commented that rates were high for "a woman your age," she asked, "Even if I stop hang-gliding and sky-diving?"

Mark Twain suggested that wrinkles should only be where smiles have been. If we have to have wrinkles, why not have them from smiles, rather than from scowls?

Free to Use Your Experience

What do you have that younger people don't? The answer is *experience,* and it's a terrific advantage. What have you learned that you could pass along to others?

A woman who struggled for years with her tendency toward child abuse channeled her energy into writing a book on this topic. Another at age forty-five was sixty pounds overweight, in the grips of a dangerous prescription drug habit and a nicotine addiction, fed by over three packs of Camels a day. Today, in her fifties, she is slim, trim, and teaches at a center for women who are overweight and defeated.

"After all, I've been there," she explains. "I can tell them, 'I've been fat. I've been sick. Do you think the Blue Fairy came along and zapped me and suddenly made me well?' "

Free to Try Something New

A seminar on "The Healing Power of Laughter and Play" suggested making a list of twenty activities that would be fun to do, ten of which cost less than five dollars. It might be interesting to stretch yourself further and come up with twenty activities you've never done before but would like to try.

Do you yearn to scuba dive? Play the piano? Make a quilt? Do woodwork? Would you like to visit that church whose pastor you've heard on the radio? Go to the Holy Land? Enjoy a sunrise picnic breakfast on the beach or in the woods?

Perhaps you will look for serene pursuits. Or you might be more like a ninety-six-year-old woman we heard about who has a keen appetite for adventure. Each birthday, starting with her ninetieth, she did something exciting that she'd never done before. One year she rode a motorcycle at seventy-five miles an hour. Another, she took a trip in a hot-air balloon, ascending from the church parking lot, with the entire congregation on hand to cheer her onward and upward.

It might be that God has given you a secret desire, something which was never before possible. A retiree in Bev's community recently fulfilled a long-standing dream by moving to New Guinea to work with Wycliffe Bible translators. Another had always wanted to be a clown and now ministers to patients of all ages in hospitals.

Take the time to start your list. If you're married, ask your husband to make one, too. You may be surprised and pleased to find that some of your secret desires are identical.

Free to Learn Something New

Why not combine the wisdom of experience with a new avenue of learning? Don't buy the lie that your brain can't handle it. If it's a formal classroom situation, it may take a while to redevelop study habits, but that's true of young people who leave school for a while, too. A recent study indicates that people who are involved in midlife mental exercise are more likely to retain mental skills in later years. Perhaps now is the time to learn to speak a new language. Or maybe you've been thinking of studying Greek to understand the New Testament better.

Possibly you can equip yourself to do a job better. Candy, who found herself frequently approached by troubled young men and women seeking her counsel, decided she needed to develop specific skills. "I knew it was helpful to them just to be listened to. But there would come a point when they needed to regroup and act. I wasn't sure how to help them direct themselves. So I took a course in counseling for lay people."

Free to Rekindle Old Interests

Is there something you loved doing in the past, but abandoned because of the time crunch? Maybe now there *is* time to pursue it once again.

As a child, Mary always loved to write poetry. But with five children, she found it impossible to find the moments to think of new ideas, much less to write them down. Now with her children raised, she's returned to that first love. And she's also interviewing her elderly parents to write a family history that she can pass along to her offspring.

Audrey was a child prodigy violinist. She decided, however, that a career as a concert violinist, with the obligatory travel, would not mix well with marriage. A few years ago, she began practicing again, and she recently delighted a music study group with a minirecital.

And Carol, whose great-grandmother taught her lace tatting, decided to resume the art. To her surprise, a whole new generation of young women wanted to learn to make these decorative trims for dresses, table linens, and handkerchiefs.

What have you enjoyed in the past? Whether it's sewing, speaking, golf, teaching, singing, or an in-depth Bible study, now you very likely have time and energy to do it again.

Free to Pursue a Career

Perhaps you already have a career to which you can now give more of yourself, or possibly you'd like to begin working. After all, the virtuous woman of Proverbs 31 was a doer who worked outside her home. And think of all the women in history who achieved greatness during their post-menopausal years: Golda Meir, Eleanor Roosevelt, Mother Teresa, Margaret Thatcher, Grandma Moses, Pearl Buck.

Colleges and universities are full of women with graying hair, equipping themselves to enter or reenter the job market. Many employers tell us that the more mature woman is highly desirable, because she's so much more dependable than the flighty neophyte or the mother of young children with her frequent family emergencies.

A number of women find that the volunteer work they did during their child-raising years is a definite plus on their resumés. One, who was chairman of some two thousand women in her county's philharmonic committees, now works for a community association management company. Interacting with the volunteer members of the community's various boards of directors is a natural for her, after all her experience with philharmonic volunteers. Another woman, who held the same philharmonic office, is now cultural director for a nearby town.

Joyce, who was born in England and has traveled extensively in Europe and Africa, attended night school courses while her children were still at home, then became a valued representative of a travel agency.

Sue was a model as a young woman and always had a flair for fashion coordination. Now she's an image consultant who helps other women use color, line, and style effectively so they can look their very best. She takes particular joy in working with her peers, who tend to be discouraged with the body and facial changes of maturing.

If you choose to work, whatever you do, don't do it simply to fill time or just to make extra money. Do something you love.

"The most important thing is to fall in love with your work," advised George Burns, still going strong at near ninety. "I love getting up in the morning because of what I do."

Free to Start New Relationships

Menopause can be a time of inertia and fatigue, a time when single women—especially those who are widowed or divorced—are not eager to reach out for new relationships. But once menopause is over and the season of renewal arrives, there's no reason to stay in the same, sometimes lonely spot. Seek out situations where you can meet new companions; join a church group, work for a political party, pursue a favorite sport. Invite a group to your home for coffee, brunch, or dinner. Remember, this is a day when it's acceptable for single women to extend invitations to men. So if there's someone you'd like to know better, by all means ask him to join you for a picnic, a play, a concert, lunch, or dinner.

Free to Care for Your Husband

When we're in the midst of menopause those of us who are married don't always do a wonderful job of keeping our husbands number one in our lives after the Lord. We tend to become preoccupied with ourselves; and, when we already feel unseasonably warm so much of the time, we may not be as enthusiastic about physical closeness as in the past.

Most of us can look back on those years and marvel at our husbands' patience. "Jeff never gave me what-can-you-expect-of-a-menopausal-woman looks, even when I was my most unreasonable or childish," one wife remembered. And another praised her spouse for "being truly protective, wisely helping me say no to requests and demands which he sensed were more than I could handle at that time."

Even if our husbands weren't paragons of patience and encouragement, we should be grateful for their staying power during a critical time for a marriage; some don't survive. Postmenopausal years can be a special time of giving back to them, and, with children gone or at least needing less from us, it's also easier to concentrate on doing for our husbands.

After Erma Bombeck's kids moved out, she threw the trough away and bought two tulip-shaped place mats. We, too, can make dinners a little more gracious for "just the two of us." We can all help by keeping a light hand and a tender touch at home to contrast with men's pressures at work. The wife whose husband helped her say no during menopause now finds that *he's* feeling a lack of discretionary time, so she can now stand between him and additional drains on his time.

Think about what special, thoughtful acts might please your husband. If you run out of ideas, you might check to see what he's written on his "fun-to-do" list.

Free to Serve Others

In your earlier years, you gave to others, especially your children, because you had to. Certainly you wanted to, but you also felt an obligation as a parent. Now you are free to give because you choose to.

Children

"Once upon a time," one mother began, "I wondered when I'd hang up my shingle as a mother. But I've concluded the answer is never. They still seek my opinion, which, of course, delights me and they share their triumphs and disappointments."

Another mother picked up the narrative, "And just when we thought ours had flown the nest, one was back living with us while he finished college and the other decided to rent an apartment adjoining our house."

But even when offspring are not under the same roof, the truth of the matter is that, as mothers, we never stop caring. So we take chicken soup to the daughter who just suffered a miscarriage, bake our special cream puffs for our offsprings' holiday parties, and stand ready to give tea and sympathy whenever the need arises.

One mother who strikes a beautiful balance of concern without intrusion is Ann, who has eleven offspring, counting sons and daughters-in-law. Ann takes time on a regular basis to send to each of them loving, beautifully thought-out notes and cards, keeping them ever aware of her interest, esteem, and support. Her gifts to them are always sensitive to the individual: a montage of photographs for the nostalgic one, a favorite verse in her calligraphy for another, a scrapbook of press clippings from a son's campaign for state office.

If you haven't any children or if yours are far away, you might have an opportunity to parent someone else. In many churches, the out-of-college singles group is filled with young people who are far away from their own parents. A number of older women have spent many happy hours discipling or "training the younger women," as Titus 2:4 suggests.

Grandchildren

If you already have grandchildren, you don't need to be told what a very special bond of giving and taking exists between the older and younger generations. If not, perhaps you can look forward to this relaxed, nonjudgmental relationship, which can nourish both generations. Some of us have had the privilege of seeing this generous spirit as our own parents loved and watched over our children. Now we have the chance to keep that momentum flowing to our children's children. What a privilege for us to marvel in the growth and development of God's new creations, to relearn simple pleasures, and to know the power of laughter and play.

You might enjoy filling out a "Grandparent's Book" of your life remembrances, for them to have as they grow up.

But even more important, we have a unique opportunity to demonstrate to our grandchildren the faithfulness of the Lord to all generations. We can nourish their spiritual heritage, as we read to them from God's Word and share with them what it means to us and what it can mean to them. "Pass it on!" is the key phrase here. And most of all, we can let them know that we pray for them.

Some of us have the privilege of practicing the art of

grandparenting with our nieces' and nephews' children. But if you're short on opportunities to give to the very young, you might consider "adopting" a grandson and/or grand-daughter or two. We suspect you won't have to look very far to find a child waiting, perhaps right on your own block.

Parents

Now, at last, after years of taking from our parents, we can choose to give to them! Of course, we can never truly re-pay them for what they've done for us, and in most cases it's not a matter of giving them *things*. "I'm past the age of ac-quisition," one parent bluntly told her children. What we *can* give them, and what they desire most, is ourselves. How they yearn for our time, for us to listen to them and feel with them.

A daughter recently chided her eighty-seven-year-old father for his impatience with his housekeeper. You don't understand!" he exclaimed. He was giving the daughter, she suddenly realized, a long-delayed replay of her recurring teenage theme to him."He was right," she realized. "I *didn't* understand his frustration over his lack of mobility and inde-pendence and over his housekeeper's mental slowness. I needed to truly listen to him and to look for solutions. And I needed, too, to listen to his reminiscences. I learned not to interrupt with 'You've told that story before, Dad,' but to en-courage him with, 'And then what happened? And how did you feel about that?' "

One elderly parent expressed this same desire for com-panionship when a son came to visit from two thousand miles away and asked, "What can I do for you, Mom?" Her reply: "Just be here."

Some of us may not have experienced perfect parent-ing, and perhaps we still harbor some resentments from those early days. If this is true of you, we urge you to free yourself from these crippling emotions, by seeking God's for-giveness for any bitterness in your heart and by forgiving your parents. Do everything you can to build a new relationship while you still can.

Of course, there's also an unending list of thoughtful things to do with and for parents who live nearby. Those in retirement communities love to go where they can watch children at play, or simply visit a shopping mall where they can people-watch a broad age span. The possibilities of places to take them are as broad as the parents' fields of interest, from church to concerts to restaurants or, probably best of all, to our homes for a meal of their favorite foods.

If we live some distance from our parents, regular, long distance phone calls are a must. But don't forget the staying power of a letter. Many of us have found letters we wrote years and years ago tucked away in our parents' desk drawers, worn from unfolding and refolding.

Another important gift we can give our parents is to build them up spiritually. Whether they're longtime believers or don't yet know the Lord, this is probably their greatest need. At an age when they're most fragile physically, they often face some of life's cruelest adjustments: loss of a spouse, moving from the family home, physical impairment. It's important to share our faith with them and to pray with them and for them. And it's equally important to assure them that, though they may no longer be necessary in terms of our physical welfare, they still have a vital role: to pray for *us*.

Community

All through this chapter, we've touched on ideas that involve giving of ourselves to others. But we'd be remiss if we didn't point to volunteerism. What keeps hospital thrift shops, soup kitchens, art museums, school enrichment programs, church projects and a host of other worthy causes going and thriving? People who give of their time and talents, of course!

There is simply no excuse for a woman's feeling bored

or wondering what to do with her day when the needs for time and talent are so great. Think about your gifts, those things that you do easily and well. Then match them with a need that truly captures your heart. If you don't know quite how to begin, see if your community has a volunteer bureau. Read your newspaper for information on which organizations do what. Make a phone call and ask, "Can you use me?" The answer, you may be sure, will be yes!

Free to Serve the Lord in New Ways

Adéle had a mastectomy twenty years ago. A few years later, cancer appeared again. Hospitalized for a hysterectomy, she *knew* she would be healed. She awoke from the anesthetic with Psalm 116:12-13 echoing through her mind: "What shall I render to the LORD For all his benefits toward me? I will take up the cup of salvation, And call upon the name of the LORD."

That is exactly what she did. She resigned her teaching job and she and her husband, Will, dedicated each room of their home to the Lord. Through the years, they welcomed hundreds of people to stay with them, sometimes for a few days, often for months. Students, families of patients undergoing treatment at the nearby hospital, to all of them, Adéle gave friendship and hospitality, often lifting "the cup of salvation" for them. A few years ago, they sold the family home and bought a much larger structure so they could minister to even more people. They call it the "House of God's Goodness."

What will *you* render to the Lord for all his goodness to you? In what new ways might you serve him? Perhaps your gift, like Adéle's, is hospitality, and you can receive visitors who come from out of town to your church or perhaps provide the setting for a Bible study or youth group. Or maybe you can offer always-needed help in the Sunday school. You needn't be a retired school teacher to be enormously effective.

Is it possible there's a ministry for you in your own neighborhood, in a retirement home, a hospital, or a prison? Or do you have a professional skill, in such fields as law, finance, architecture, music, which you could volunteer to your church or another needy body? Perhaps you're ready to find a new need, a cause in our hurting world and to wage your own war for truth and righteousness.

Think about it. Pray about it. Give yourself with a heartfelt, "Here am I!" to the Lord. Be open to new ways to glorify Him. Do it as a thanks offering for all He has done for you.

Free to Grow in Your Knowledge and Love of Him

If you're a mother, you undoubtedly remember the days when the children were very young and you tried to find time to pray and read your Bible before everyone was up. However the earlier you rose, the earlier *they* wakened. Perhaps you longed for the concentration of John Wesley's mother, who, with a huge houseful of children, simply pulled her apron over her head to pray.

Chances are you now can spend blocks of quality time with the Lord. Here's your opportunity to work your way through the entire Bible with a guide such as *The Daily Walk*. Or, you may enjoy reading a book of daily meditations, such as Charles Spurgeon's *Morning and Evening*.

Perhaps this is the time to find an in-depth Bible study, which will challenge you to dig and question and discuss what you discover. Or, you might like to do your own topical study, choosing a subject such as "getting organized" or "learning patience" or "God as my defender." Consult a Strong's Concordance to find the verses on this topic, and then read a passage of Scripture daily. If you haven't a support group already, why not gather together regularly with four or five other women, so you can share and express concerns and pray for one another?

The closing words of the great Passion chorale, "O Sacred Head, Now Wounded," might well be our ongoing prayer: "Lord, let me never, never outlive my love for thee!"

Whatever you choose to do with your time, we urge that you do it wholeheartedly, as if it all depends on you, while all the while you know that it depends on Him. And always see it as a witness, a reflection of His love and glory. A wise pastor once told us, "A job well done *is* a witness!"

The temptation, of course, will be to try to do too much. When Mary realized her nest was about to empty, she pondered aloud what she would do with her time. And her husband, who knew her very well, replied, "It will be just like the shelves I build for you. The more I build, the more you find to fill them."

As you think about what you'd like to do, try not to fill your "shelves" to overflowing. Instead, ask yourself two questions: Will I pull in and only do for me, or will I choose also to give to others? Will I do a lot, or will I do one or two things really well?

A recurring theme in the teaching of Anne Ortlund, who wrote *Disciplines of the Beautiful Woman*, is to "eliminate and concentrate." The most effective Christians, she points out, are the least complicated, those who are not trying to be several selves. She urges, "Discover what is the irreduceable minimum for you, the one thing you must have, the reason God created you. You have one great purpose in life, and God's great commissions are simple. Find that one thing."[1]

Most of us are happiest when we do not allow ourselves to be fragmented but find a single, central focus. What will it be for you? Seek it with all your heart. A third or a half of your life is a terrible thing to waste!

A LAST WORD

We hope this book has given you a sense of informed optimism and confidence in dealing with your climacteric years.

It is our wish, too, that this book may be used in study groups to clarify the individual variations of menopause and to stimulate discussion of the changes during this time of transition.

In organizing the material, Orene has found it strengthening to delve into the problems and solutions that are unique to menopause, not just as a physician, but as a woman looking forward to her own climacteric.

"I do a great deal of wondering about what my experience will be, as I pass through this stage of life with so many women," Orene says. "Partly, this stems from my empathy for my patients. (I often wonder if I will cope as well as many of them.) But it's also because I believe that *preparation* is absolutely critical to a smooth passage through a stage of life or a new life situation."

As a gynecologist and surgeon, Orene realizes she will not be able to carry on with her work schedule if she experiences excessive bleeding for a prolonged period of time or continuous hot flushes. Thus hysterectomy or hormone replacement therapy may become a necessity for her.

In addition, she has watched a grandmother live to the age of ninety-six, with increasing curvature of the spine and bending of the thorax. Finally she couldn't even read a book, because she could not raise her head sufficiently to focus on the pages. She also suffered a fractured hip.

Thus Orene, in her forties, is supplementing her calcium intake and participating in such bone-stressing exercises as jogging and aerobics. Estrogen replacement therapy may be indicated for her at menopause.

"How happy I am," Orene states, "that my menopause will be in the 1980s, rather than even the sixties or seventies! We are so fortunate in this decade to have good, sound information on hormone replacement therapy, osteoporosis, and a multitude of resources to promote good physical, emotional, and spiritual health in the climacteric.

"As stewards of our bodies, we all have a responsibility

to learn all we can, to take this knowledge seriously, and to use it effectively to help us make a change for the better."

NOTES

Chapter 1: Change for the Better

1. Quotations from "All in the Family" used by permission of Tandem Productions from the teleplay written by Bert Styler. Tandem Productions. All rights reserved.

Chapter 6: What about My Sex Life?

1. Quotation from Dr. William Masters cited in Wendy Cooper's *No Change* (Tiptree, Essex, England: Anchor Press, 1983), p. 73.
2. Edward M. Brecher et. al., *Love, Sex and Aging* (Mount Vernon, New York: Consumers Union, 1984), p. 17.
3. Ann Landers in *The Los Angeles Times*, February 18, 1985.
4. Quotation from David Augsburger cited in *For Women Only*, eds. Evelyn and J. Allan Petersen (Wheaton, Illinois: Tyndale, 1982), p. 140.
5. Tim and Beverly LaHaye, *The Act of Marriage* (Grand Rapids, Michigan: Zondervan, 1976), p. 312.
6. Robert Butler and Myrna Lewis, *Sex After Sixty* (Boston: G. K. Hall and Company, 1977), pp. 233-239.

Chapter 9: "I'm Just So Emotional!"

1. Evelyn Keyes, "Wrinkles That Matter," Los Angeles Time Calendar, February 17, 1985.
2. G. Mitchell, *Human Sex Difference* (New York: Van Nostrand Reinhold Company, 1981), p. 166.

Chapter 11: The Shaping of Attitudes

1. Estelle Fuch, *The Second Season* (U.S.A.: The Anchor Press, 1977), p. 172.
2. Ibid., p. 173.
3. Ibid., p. 174.

Chapter 14: Celebrating Your Freedom

1. Cited from Anne Ortlund's *Disciplines of the Beautiful Woman* and from her teaching in a Bible class at Mariners Church, Newport Beach, California.

BIBLIOGRAPHY

Chapter 1: Change for the Better

Notelovitz. Morris. (1982). Climacteric medicine and climacteric science. *Menopause Update, 1* (1), 2-4.

Williams, Charlotte. (1982). A woman's perspective...menopause. *Menopause Update, 1* (1).16-17.

Chapter 2: What Is Menopause?

Jones, Howard W., and Jones, Georgeanna Seegar. (1981). *Novak's Textbook of Gynecology* (10th ed.). Baltimore: Williams and Willkins Company.

Sciarra, John H. (ed.). (1984). *Gynecology and Obstetrics.* Philadelphia: Harper and Row.

Yussman, Marvin A., Taymor, Melvin L., et al. (1970). Serum levels of follicle-stimulating hormone, luteinizing hormone and plasma progestins correlated with human ovulation. *Fertility and Sterility. 21* (2). 119-125.

Zinca, Victoria. (1970). The endocrinology, biochemistry, and cytomorphology of the menses. *The Woman Physician, 25* (11), 697-704.

Chapter 3: Is Anyone Else Here Feeling Warm?

Gambrell, R.D., Jr., et al. (1983). Decreased incidence of breast cancer in postmenopausal estrogen-progestogen users. *Obstetrics and Gynecology, 62,* 435-443.

Gold, Jay J., Josimovich, John B. (1980). *Gynecologic Endocrinology.* Hagerstown, Maryland: Harper and Row.

Judd, Howard L., Cleary, Robert E. (1981). Estrogen replacement therapy. *Obstetrics and Gynecology, 58,* 267-275.

Kistner, R.W. (1971). *Gynecology Principles and Practice* (2nd ed.). Chicago: Yearbook Medical Publishers.

Molnar, George W. (1975). Body temperatures during menopausal hot flashes. *Journal of Applied Physiology, 38* (3), 499-503.

Norris, Ronald V., and Sullivan, Colleen. (1983). *PMS Premenstrual Syndrome.* New York: Rawson Associates.

Notelovitz, Morris. (1983). Estrogens, lipids, and coronary heart disease-a hypothesis. *Midlife Wellness, 1* (3), 38-41.

Notelovitz, Morris, and Ware, Marsha. (1982). *Stand Tall.* Gainsville, Florida: Triad Publishing Company, Inc.

Wied, George L. (ed.). (1983). Premenstrual tension: An invitational symposium. *The Journal of Reproductive Medicine, 28* (8), 503-538.

Chapter 4: Coping with the Changes

Hammond, Charles B., and Maxson, Wayne S. (1982). Current status of estrogen therapy for the menopause. *Fertility and Sterility, 37* (1), 5-25.

Laufer, Larry R., and Erlik, Yohanan, et al. (1982). Effect of clonidine on hot flashes in postmenopausal women. *Obstetrics and Gynecology, 60* (5), 583-586.

Norris, Ronald V., and Sullivan, Colleen. (1983). *PMS Premenstrual Syndrome.* New York: Rawson Associates.

Ware, Marsha. (1982). Can vitamin E help control hot flashes? *Menopause Update 1* [1], 33.

Wied, George L. (ed.). (1983). Premenstrual tension: An invitational symposium. *The Journal of Reproductive Medicine, 28* (8), 503-538.

Chapter 5: Is Estrogen for You?

ACOG Technical Bulletin. (1983) *Estrogen replacement therapy* (Bulletin No. 70). Washington, D.C.: American College of Obstetricians and Gynecologists.

ACOG Technical Bulletin. (1983) *Epidemiology and diagnosis of breast disease* (Bulletin No. 71). Washington, D.C.: American College of Obstetricians and Gynecologists.

ACOG Technical Bulletin. (1984) *Carcinoma of the endometrium* (Bulletin No. 76). Washington, D.C.: American College of Obstetricians and Gynecologists.

Campbell, S., McQueen, J., et al. (1978). The modifying effect of progestogen on the response of the post-menopausal endometrium to exogenous estrogens. *Postgraduate Medical Journal, 54:* Supplement 2, 59-64.

Deutsch, S., et al. (1981). Comparison between degree of systemic absorption of vaginally and orally administered estrogens at different dose levels in postmenopausal women. *American Journal of Obstetrics and Gynecology, 139,* 967-968.

Druzin, Maurice (ed.). (1984). Estrogens after menopause: How do you keep your balance? *Data Centrum Obstetrics and Gynecology Supplement, 1* (4), 2-7.

Gambrell, R.D., Jr., et al. (1983). Decreased incidence of breast cancer in postmenopausal estrogen-progestogen users. *Obstetrics and Gynecology, 62,* 435-443.

Greenblatt, Robert B. (1982). The menopause—past, present, and future. *Menopause Update, 1* (1), 10-14.

Gurtman, Angel Issac, Andrack, Juan Angel, et al. (1957). Long-acting estrogens in amenorrhea and menopause. *Obstetrics and Gynecology, 10* (3), 261-265.

Knopp, Robert H. (guest ed.). (1984). Oral contraceptives and lipid metabolism. *New Perspectives on Oral Contraception, 1* (3).

Martin, Purvis, Greaney, Martin O., et al. (1984). Estradiol, estrone, and gonadotropin levels after use of vaginal estrogen. *Obstetrics and Gynecology, 63* (4), 441-444.

Mashchak, C. Ann, Lobo, Rogerio A., et al. (1982). Comparison of pharmacodynamic properties of various estrogen formulations. *American Journal of Obstetrics and Gynecology, 144* (5), 511-518.

Mastroianni, Luigi. (ed.). (1984). The medical challenge of menopause. *OBG Diagnosis, 3* (1), 1-8.

Nachtigall, L.E., Nachtigall, R.H., et al. (1979). Estrogen replacement therapy I: A ten-year prospective study in the relationship to osteoporosis. *Obstetrics and Gynecology, 53,* 277.

Petitti, Diana B. (1983). Menopausal estrogens and vascular disease. *Midlife Wellness, 1* (3), 9-12.

Ravnikar, V.A. (1983). When your patient faces menopause. *Patient Care, 17,* 91-117.

Sciarra, John H. (ed.). (1984). *Gynecology and Obstetrics.* Philadelphia: Harper and Row.

Sipinen, S., and Lahteenmaki, P. (1980). Steroid and gonadotropin profiles in menopausal women on three different oral replacement regimens. *Annals of Clinical Research, 12,* 282-287.

Wren, Barry G., and Routledge, Anthony D. (1983). The effect of type and dose of estrogen on the blood pressure of postmenopausal women. *Maturitas, 5.* 135-142.

Chapter 6: What about My Sex Life?

Bachmann, Gloria, Leiblum, Sandra, et al. (1984). Vaginal atrophy in postmenopausal dysparunia. *The Female Patient, 9,* 118-127.

Brencher, Edward M., et al. (1984). *Love, Sex, and Aging: A*

Consumers Union Report. Mount Vernon, N.Y.: Consumers Union.

Butler, Robert N. and Lewis, Myrna I. (1977). *Sex after Sixty.* Boston: G.K. Hall and Co.

A Clinical Guide to the Menopause and the Postmenopause. (1968). New York: Ayerst Laboratories, 45-49.

Gray, Madeline. (1967). *The Changing Years.* New York: Doubleday.

Greenhill and Friedman. (1974). *Biological Principles and Modern Practice of Obstetrics and Gynecology.* Philadelphia: Saunders.

LaHaye, Tim and Beverly. (1976). *The Act of Marriage.* Grand Rapids, Mich.: Zondervan Publishing House.

Petersen, Evelyn R. and Petersen, J. Allan (eds.). (1982). *For Women Only.* Wheaton, Ill.: Tyndale.

Rubin, Isadore. (1965). *Sexual Life after Sixty.* New York: Basic Books.

Shedd, Charlie, and Shedd, Martha. (1979). *Celebration in the Bedroom.* Waco, Texas: Word Books.

Shedd, Charlie. (1968). *The Stork Is Dead.* Waco, Texas: Word Books.

Sheehy, Gail. (1974). *Passages.* New York: Bantum Books.

Vincent, Clark E. (1968). *Human Sexuality in Medical Education and Practice.* Springfield, Illinois: Thomas.

Woods, Nancy Fulgate. (1975). *Human Sexuality in Health and Illness.* St. Louis: C.V. Mosby.

Chapter 7: How to Avoid Dowager's Hump

Donaldson, C.L., Hulley, S.B., et al. (1970). Effect of prolonged bed rest on bone mineral content. *Metabolism, 19,* 1071-1084.

Krause, M.V., and Mahan, L.K. (1979). *Food, Nutrition, and Diet Therapy.* Philadelphia: W.B. Sanders Co.

Mack, P.B., La Chance, P.A., et al. (1967). Bone demineralization of foot and hand of Gemini-Titan IV, V, and VII astronauts during orbital flight. *American Journal Roentgen. 100,* 503-511.

Nachtigall, L.E., Nachtigall, R.H., et al. (1979). Estrogen replacement therapy I: A ten-year prospective study in the relationship to osteoporosis. *Obstetrics and Gynecology, 53,* 277.

Notelovitz, Morris, and Ware, Marsha. (1982). *Journal of Ameri-*

can Medical Association, 252 (6), 799-802.

Ravnikar, V.A. (1983). When your patient faces menopause. Patient Care, 17, 91-117.

Richart, Ralph. (guest ed.). (1984). Osteoporosis and its relationship to estrogen. Contemporary OB/GYN, 201-224.

Riggs, B. Lawrence, et al. (1982). Effect of the fluoride/calcium regimen on vertebral fracture occurrence in postmenopausal osteoporosis. New England Journal of Medicine, 306 (8), 446-450.

Ross, R.K., Paganini-Hill, A., et al. (1980). A case-control study of menopausal estrogen therapy and breast cancer. Journal of American Medical Association, 243, 1635.

Smith, Everett L. (1984). The role of exercise in prevention of osteoporosis. Midpoint: Counseling Women through the Menopause, 1 (2), 3-6.

Smith, Everett L., Reddan, William, et al. (1981). Physical activity and calcium modalities for bone mineral increase in aged women. Medicine and Science in Sports and Exercise. 13 (1), 60-64.

Smith, Everett L., Smith, Patricia E., et al. (1984). Bone involution decrease in exercising middle-aged women. Calcified Tissue International, 36, S129-S138.

Chapter 8: Three Ounces of Prevention

Cooper, Wendy. (1983). No Change. Tiptree, Essex, Great Britain: Anchor Press Ltd.

Hall, Deborah C., Goldstein, Mark Kane, and Stein, Gerald. (1977). Progress in manual breast examination. Cancer, 40 (1), 364-370.

Isenman, Albert W. (ed.). Quality Assurance in Obstetrics and Gynecology. Washington, D.C.: American College of Obstetrics and Gynecologists.

Jones, Howard W., and Jones, Georgeanna Seegar. (1981). Novak's textbook of Gynecology (10th ed.). Baltimore: Williams and Wilkins Company.

Mattingly, Richard F. (1977). Telinde's Operative Gynecology (5th ed.). Philadelphia: J. B. Lippencott Company.

Pennypacker, H.S., Bloom, H.S., et al. (1982). Toward an effective technology of instruction in breast self-examination. International Journal of Mental Health, 11 (3), 98-116.

Chapter 9: I'm Just So Emotional!

Mastroianni, Luigi. (ed.). (1984). The medical challenge of menopause. *OBG Diagnosis, 3* (1), 1-8.

Mitchell, G. (1981). *Human Sex Difference: A Primatologist's Perspective.* New York: Van Nostrand Reinhold Co.

Ross, R.K., Paganini-Hill, A., et al. (1980). A case-control study of menopausal estrogen therapy and breast cancer. *Journal of American Medical Association, 243,* 1635.

Yost, Murray A., Jr. (1984). Psychology of the climacteric. In S. S. Sciarra (ed.). *Gynecology and Obstetrics* (pp. 2-4). Philadelphia: Harper and Row.

Chapter 11: The Shaping of Attitudes

Aron, Nancy, et al. (1981). *A Time to Reap.* Baltimore: University Press.

du Toit, Bryan. (1984). Menopause—a cross-cultural perspective. *Midlife Wellness, 1* (4), 66-67.

Flint, Marcha P. (1982). First symposium on the menopause. *Menopause Update, 1* (1), 23.

Fuchs, Estelle. (1977). *The Second Season.* U.S.A.: The Anchor Press.

Mead, Margaret. (1949). *Male and Female.* New York: William Morrow & Co.

Mitchell, G. (1981). *Human Sex Difference—A Primatologist's Perspective.* New York: Van Nostrand Reinhold Co.

Wright, Ann L. (1982). Variation in Navajo menopause: Toward an explanation. In Ann M. Voda, Myra Dinnerstein, and Sheryl R. O'Donnell (Eds.), *Changing Perspectives on Menopause* (pp. 84-99). Austin, Texas: University of Texas Press.

INDEX